# Same Time... Same Station

A Memoir:
An Epic Love and Life Story

By
Cecily Kohlsaat Hitchcock

**Same Time... Same Station**



ISBN 978-1506-903-57-6 PRINT
ISBN 978-1506-903-58-3 EBOOK

LCCN 2016960471

November 2016

Published and Distributed by
First Edition Design Publishing, Inc.
P.O. Box 20217, Sarasota, FL 34276-3217
www.firsteditiondesignpublishing.com

*To my beloved Husband,*
*Peter Tilden Hitchcock,*
*who wanted me to write*
*this book.*

## Table of Contents


Introduction ..... 1
The Secret of Our Lasting Marriage ..... 3

**Part One: Our Beginnings** ..... 5
- Early Years ..... 5
- How We Met ..... 13
- Our Courtship ..... 17
- Meeting My Parents ..... 24
- The Slip Up ..... 34

**Part Two: Wedding Belles** ..... 35
- The Trip to Bronxville ..... 35
- The Proposal ..... 39
- Wedding Plans ..... 44
- The Duck and I ..... 47

**Part Three: Married Life** ..... 53
- Keeping in Touch ..... 53
- The Trip to Bermuda ..... 61
- Love Letters from India ..... 68
- Joining Peter in Europe ..... 78

**Part Four: Life Challenges** ..... 89
- Moving to Bronxville ..... 89
- Off to Houston, Texas ..... 102
- The Accident: The Trip to Heaven ..... 111
- Peter's Lawsuit ..... 115

**Part Five: Going Forward** ..... 119
- The Diagnosis ..... 119
- Unexpected Happenings ..... 126
- Early Signs of Parkinson's Disease ..... 129
- Accepting Help ..... 136

**Part Six: A Rocky Road Ahead** ..... 141
- Reminiscing ..... 141
- The Last Straw ..... 145
- Home at Last ..... 150
- The Turning Point ..... 153

**Part Seven: Acceptance** ..... 165
- An Unexpected Move ..... 165

The Quagmire of Dementia ........................................ 168
Just You and Me ........................................ 172

**Epilogue: Reaching Out** ........................................ 178

Acknowledgements ........................................ 185

# Introduction

Several years ago my late Husband, Peter Tilden Hitchcock, asked me to write a book, which I have named, "Same Time…Same Station," sharing our story of profound love and strong partnership that grew deeper and stronger, as we lived through life's challenges for the fifty-four years we shared. No one should endure such overwhelming and devastating afflictions as we did. It was our strong love that got us through. We became inseparable, faithful to each other and trusting, always finding joy in what we were doing together. We just wanted to be with one another, eventually becoming soul mates. I believe the reader will find our story inspiring, uplifting, and even challenging.

Peter once told me: "There's a reason for my having Parkinson's…to help people cope with the disease. More research should be done, as Parkinson's disease is prevalent. Too much money and time are being spent on other diseases. We are spiritual, Ceci. I accept my getting the disease, because I know we will be together again one day." He always hoped that in the future his rigidity could be stopped!

Peter was Special Counsel of the International Division of Allied Chemical Corporation and traveled extensively. We stayed close during these separations by writing love letters to each other, which I'd like to share.

Eventually we became caregivers to one another, but we never felt as such. We wanted to take care of each other both during my accident and four surgeries, and his battle with Parkinson's disease. We lived each day to the fullest, our love bringing in sunshine and hope.

"Same Time…Same Station" is a tribute to all caregivers and their loved ones. I found that, if planned well, caregiving doesn't have to be dreaded and exhausting. There are, of course, exceptions depending upon the circumstances, the loved one, and the illness. I write not from a medical point of view but from personal experience that lasted fourteen years. At the end, validation is absolutely necessary to have a peaceful, less stressful relationship; that is, forget yourself and your feelings and enter into the world of your loved one. Do not argue! Try to do research as much as possible to learn about your loved one's illness to better understand what he or she is going through.

Research well Independent and Assisted Living, or a Skilled Nursing Facility versus Home Care, before making a decision. Our only regret is that we had to enter a facility. We had Long Term Care which we paid for eleven years. Our agent advised us that it would be too costly. We wish we hadn't listened to him and paid the extra money each month. Peter would have preferred staying in our home among familiar surroundings.

I would like to take this opportunity to say "thank you" to all those who took care of Peter.

Some names have been changed for privacy, and if I quote anyone without recognition, please forgive me. A correction will be made in the next edition.

# The Secret of Our Lasting Marriage

Our Love was a gift,
It was beautiful.
We believed in each other.
It was fresh energy.

During our Courtship,
We became inseparable,
Always having fun,
Sharing,
Giving,
Being unselfish,
And passionate.
We became best friends.

In our Marriage,
We were devoted to each other.
We were honest,
Trusting,
Compromising,
Respectful,
Understanding,
And forgiving.
We became soul mates.

Raising our Children,
We were partners,
Finding time together,
Loving each other.
Through thick and thin,
We communicated,
Shared,
With patience,
Teaching,
And discipline.

During Illness,
We were loyal to each other,
Caring,
Compassionate,
Kind,
Validating,
Having hope
With faith,
And finding Joy
In each day we shared.

Our Love was a gift!

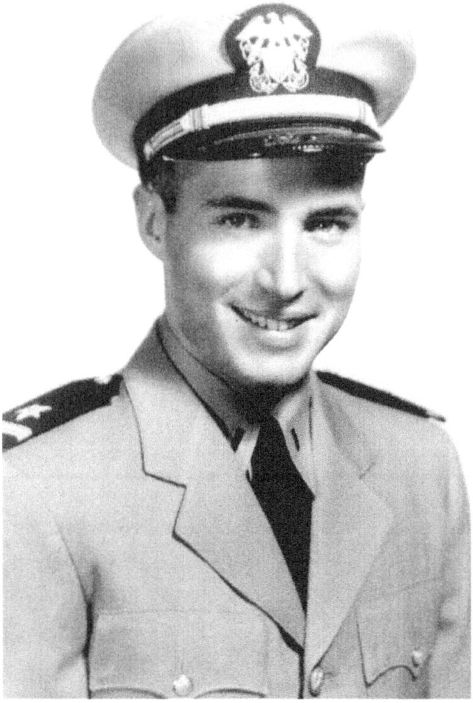

Lt. Peter Tilden Hitchcock in England during Korean War, 1953-1955

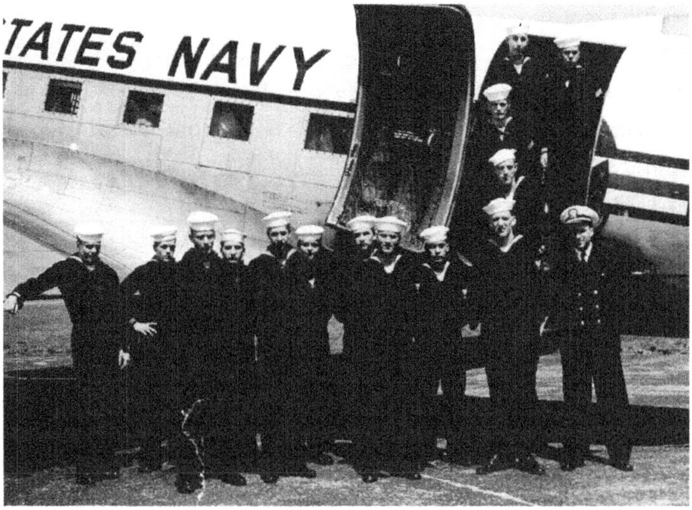


Peter with his crew, 1954

# Part One: Our Beginnings

## Early Years

Peter had a happy childhood living in Bronxville, New York with his parents, two sisters and a brother. His father was a brilliant lawyer, a partner of Chadbourne, Parke, Whiteside and Wolff in New York City.

After eighth grade, Peter's parents decided to send him off to boarding school, Phillips Exeter Academy in Exeter, New Hampshire, to further his education as he was extremely bright. He became a scholar there, adored Exeter, and enjoyed lacrosse and football. In 1949, he graduated Summa Cum Laude and picked Princeton University in Princeton, New Jersey, over Annapolis and Dartmouth, where his father graduated, Class of 1919.

Princeton offered Officer's Candidate School. Upon graduating Cum Laude in 1953, he served in the Korean War for the United States Navy. From 1950-1955, the war was fought by North Korea and China against the United Nations forces and the United States. Peter was released from active duty with an Honorable Discharge having attained the rank of Lieutenant, Senior Grade. He had been stationed in London, England which he loved.

Peter never talked about his experiences with the Navy. He was very secretive but said that some of his missions were quite dangerous. He did, however, tell me that a wave had crashed over the entire United States' ship as he traveled to England. "I wasn't afraid at all," he told me. I quote two letters that he wrote to his mother:

27 September 1953

"Dear Mommy:

The trip over was pretty rough, but a lot of fun. Several crewmen and passengers suffered broken bones due to the rolling of the ship, so I gather it was the toughest crossing the United States has made to date.

The Navy sent a car to take us to a hotel they had reserved for us. Since, I have moved, with the other Ensign, Bob Trezciak, to Dolphin Square, where we've eaten at the embassy, at the other end of Grosvenor Square from our building. There is also an officer's club, which serves meals. Once in the apartment (only for 2 months, however) we'll do our own cooking. This is very important, since we'll be standing watches at odd hours, getting off at times when restaurants are closed.

We have Navy stores on Grosvenor Square for most things, food and clothing included. Haircuts and shoeshines are provided free.

We've had beautifully warm and sunny weather to date, although it has just started to rain. The fog isn't due for another month or so, fortunately.

Let me know how all is going; this has to be short since I'm trying to get everybody tonite.

Love,

Peter"

October 7, 1953

"Dear Mommy:

I'm very sorry to have caused you so much worry. Your first cablegram reached me last Monday, as I had been sent to French Morocco on a courier run the preceding week.

I should say, however, that I wish you wouldn't worry any more. The nature of my work is such that I won't always be able to keep in constant touch with you, although I generally will be able to do so. At any rate, the Navy will notify you immediately if I should ever be hurt in any accident.

Love,

Peter"

From his letters, I learned that he loved the theatre. He would review the English plays and report his findings to his parents. The plays would eventually end up in New York City.

Upon returning to the States, he continued his education at Columbia Law School in New York City, Class of 1959. This is where we met. I was a first year student at St. Luke's School of Nursing, now St. Luke's-Roosevelt Hospital.

As for me, I had a rough and unhappy childhood. We moved nine times in eleven years finally settling in Old Greenwich, Connecticut. My grandparents stepped in whenever necessary and took care of us in their home in Princeton, New Jersey. My father, a graduate of Princeton University, class of 1931, was a talented piano player, who played by ear. He fell back on this hobby, earning money when he would lose a job. Gradually he became a drifter, unable to stay employed, and eventually became an alcoholic. When he drank he became abusive, beating my mother. He would pass out on top of me as I slept at night forcing me to sleep with my sister in her double bed. She slept at one end and I at the bottom. My father left us alone but not my older sister. He would pick up her mattress when she was fast asleep and throw her on the floor. She would climb down the Wisteria vine that climbed up onto the porch, until Mother told her to come back into the house.

Once he kept the four of us: mother, my sisters, our Cocker Spaniel, Taffy, and me locked in a room, swinging a gun around, drunk and threatening us. Mother was able to leave the room and retrieve another bottle of Bourbon which knocked him unconscious. We were nine, eleven and thirteen years old.

I remember the police and the ambulance that took my father to Stamford Hall, Stamford, Connecticut, in a strait jacket. I remember visiting him with my sisters and hearing the words

"Ceci...Ceci, please give me a drink, just a little one."

On a happy note, I do remember hearing on the radio, as we had no television in those days, "World War II is over." My youngest sister remembers going outdoors, finding a clear blue sky with lots of birds singing high above her.

After eighteen years of abuse, mother divorced my father in 1946 with the help of my Grandfather, William Starr Myers. As we left in the old Ford from Old Greenwich, our house was being auctioned off because of bankruptcy. We were told to take one thing that was precious to us. I took "Lucky" my monkey, and my sister took "Teddy." We were happy to be going back to Princeton to live!

Woodrow Wilson, President of the University, invited Grandfather, Dr. Myers as he was called, to join the faculty. They became friends. There is a family anecdote that mother, as an infant, was placed on Wilson's lap. She peed all over it!

Grandfather taught Political History from 1906-1943.Known as the historian of the Republican Party and of the Herbert Hoover Administration, he wrote many books such as "The Republican Party-a History" (1928), "The Hoover Administration" (1946), and a three-volume "Story of New Jersey." He served as an editor and speech writer for Hoover.

My Grandfather was a wonderful, loving person. I looked up to him as he always had time for me. He taught me so much; strength and courage, trust and love. He supported me in every way. As I played by ear, he would sit down at the piano next to me and listen to simple tunes I made up. Other times I would visit him in the library which housed hundreds of books enjoying a piece of candied ginger and listening to his stories.

I remember well Grandfather closing our bedroom windows at six am on school days each morning. He would then wind up the old Ship and Grandfather clocks downstairs. We three were extremely precious to him.

My Grandmother was just the opposite. She never left me alone, always criticizing and finding fault with everything I did or wore. I couldn't do anything right: She didn't like my clothes; my haircut was too short as she liked long hair tied back with a large bow; my skirts were too long; the perfume my Mother gave me smelled like sherry, and so forth. I remember well Grandfather's words, "Leave her alone, Margaret!" On top of this, she threw away "Lucky," my precious monkey... said it was attracting moths ... and she tossed away my box of trading cards. My younger sister and I would go door to door, as did our classmates at Miss Fine's School, asking for old decks of cards. We'd take them to school to trade. I must have had two hundred in all sorts of categories.

We lived with our grandparents for a while. Mother found a job working for a doctor, but eventually created her own catering business, "Starr Caterers." She frequently catered for the Governor at Morven in Princeton. As for us, we attended the private girl's school in Princeton. I remember well sitting and listening to the radio every night, especially "Lassie" and "Inner Sanctum" with its squeaky door. In the summer we went to the Lake Placid Club in Lake Placid, New York, with Grandmother and Grandfather. One summer we were sent to Camp Bueno in New Hampshire, but I loved Lake Placid.

I remember well the concerts given by Kate Smith and Paul Whitman. Kate Smith, well known for her version of the song "God Bless America," was a good friend of my grandparents. We were invited once to her home on the lake for tea. We travelled by boat to get there, docking in her boathouse which was attached to her residence. While Kate and my grandparents stayed inside, I, quite bored at the age of eleven, explored the outside – the hilly grounds and the edge of the serene lake.

Life must have been very difficult for Mother raising three children, yet she was able to do volunteer work as we moved about for the Junior League in Chicago (1931), in New York City (1934), in Washington, D.C. (1942), and in Greenwich, Connecticut (1946). Ironically, both my Mother and Peter's Mother were members in New York City at the same time but never met.

I do not think of the past with my Father. I have blocked the nightmares out of my mind; however, unknowingly, I lacked security and was afraid of the dark. I learned later that my experience with my Father influenced my total love commitment to my marriage. I never forgave my father, who moved to Florida, remarried, divorced and became engaged again to another woman. Daddy died of stomach cancer, never helping my mother financially to raise the three of us, unlike today when it is law!

In 1950, mother married Minot C. Morgan, Jr. who had three children of his own. Mike was the Mayor of Princeton in 1946. He then became Comptroller for The Institute of Advanced Study in Princeton working with Robert Oppenheimer. We were a happy family. Our house bustled with people coming and going. Mother and Mike loved to entertain whether it was with friends, Princeton University students, its singing group "The Nassoons," or out of town family members. They always had a good time and knew how to throw the perfect party. Mother frequently invited "The Nassoons" to our house or to Stone Harbor, New Jersey. To them she was known as "Ma Morgan." Ironically, my Grandfather Myers developed Parkinson's disease.

In 1952, my grandparents sent me to St. Mary's School and Junior College in Raleigh, North Carolina. Grandfather was so proud that a member of his family was attending a North Carolina school. He knew the area well as he spent his college years at the University of North Carolina – Chapel Hill, where he wrote the school's Alma Mater, "Hail to the Brightest Star, Hark the Sound."

I loved my three years at St. Mary's, graduating from the high school in 1953 and college in 1955. I was the only Yankee my first year. How surprised I was to learn how strong segregation was in the South – very different from life in the North: one never sat in the back of a bus, which I had done; one never mentioned the Ku Klux Klan which I had and was hushed by my friends, and bathrooms and drinking fountains were labeled "Black and White." Many people had very little respect for the black people.

Nevertheless, St. Mary's taught me so much: confidence and self-esteem, independence, responsibility, and the importance and joy of education. I received the honor of being a Hall Counselor; became active in all sports especially being pitcher for our softball team; was a journalist for The Belle which was a newspaper; danced in Orchesis; and enjoyed being an acolyte in our little Episcopal chapel.

I frequently heard from my grandmother, Mother Mabel, my father's mother. She lived in St. Louis, Missouri. I saw very little of her, but she constantly wrote letters of encouragement, giving me validation, a lift up, and sending me spending money. She was so proud of me that I had picked St. Mary's. I was her precious granddaughter but she was extremely disturbed over Daddy's behavior. I did see her, however, in Princeton many times after graduation as three of my cousins attended the University.

I remember in my second year at St. Mary's one amusing evening we had outside our West Rock dormitory- warned that we could have a panty raid sometime, we all kept unopened coke bottles just in case! That night we had peeping toms. I spotted them, telling Miss Vann who lived in the dormitory. She called the police, who told us to keep the prowlers' attention until they arrived. I and Miss Vann did just that. One was a Princeton graduate (from Michigan), so he said, and the other from Paris, France. They were soldiers from Fort Bragg! The police caught our two and found four other soldiers prowling on the campus. They, of course, were arrested, and we were praised by the school administration.

Again, in 1954, it was at St. Mary's that I met Phillip Morehouse (29), a proud owner of a baby blue and cream colored, winged tip Chevrolet. I was 18. Phillip was Vice President of the Senior Class at North Carolina State down the street from St. Mary's. We dated most weekends. He was quite a "Fred Astaire" dancer and a Brother at the Sigma Chi Fraternity. Great fun, were the Sigma Chi Sweetheart Ball and the House Party in Cherry Grove, South Carolina. Upon graduation in 1954, he accepted a job with a chemical company in South Carolina. We saw each other off and on at St. Mary's, or I would meet him in Charlotte, North Carolina. I then returned to Princeton where he visited me or I would meet him in the City. I never knew when I'd see him next. It was aggravating.

Peter, in the meantime, was dating a girl named Stacey, who lived in Bronxville, New York.

*****

During my years at St. Mary's I would spend the summers at home in Princeton. For three years I worked as a camp counselor at the Cortelyou's Day Camp outside of Princeton. Upon graduation in 1955, I again worked at the Camp, in charge of sixteen eight-year-olds. We had fun weaving straw baskets, making friendship bracelets, and doing other crafts besides swimming, having sleepovers and sing-alongs, and so forth.

There was great interest when the Camp received news that the farmer's dog next door had a litter of puppies. Would we be interested in having one? I, being a lover of animals, was the first to make an appearance along with several of my campers. We found six adorable blond puppies. The mother was a small, long-haired Golden Retriever mix and quite beautiful. I was lucky as one incredibly plump male jumped on my lap after I sat down, and licked my face. We fell in love. "I'm interested in this one. Can you hold him for me until tomorrow? I want to consult with my parents," I said.

To make a long story short, I adopted Pooh Bear, named by Mike, as he looked like a chubby, blond, roly-poly cub bear. I immediately took him for his shots and was told to buy a can of kerosene. He had tapeworms. I spent hours that afternoon helping Pooh get rid of the hammerhead worms. Needless to say, they were disgusting, but the kerosene killed them right on the spot- poor Pooh! Of course, it took a while for the lawn to recover too.

That fall, I accepted a secretarial job at D. Van Nostrand in Princeton, which I enjoyed. I taught myself how to type and took shorthand lessons in New Brunswick, New Jersey.

A year later, I had to have surgery to remove Dermoid Cysts from my ovaries, the size of grapefruits, filled with hair and teeth, a disorder that ran in the family. Pooh Bear was a constant companion.

However, having had enough of living in Princeton at twenty-three, I decided to go to St. Luke's School of Nursing in the City. This would mean I would have to leave Pooh with Mother until I could find an apartment. That saddened me. Still, I needed to change my surroundings, make new friends, and possibly meet my future husband. I certainly wouldn't meet him in Princeton! I wanted to be alive, have fun, and be loved.

*****

I'll never forget Mother's phone call one night at school, saying that Pooh had slipped and stumbled down the kitchen steps, some fifteen, early that morning and was paralyzed from the waist down. I was furious and devastated, as he was never allowed to go down those steps – only the four stairs out on the side porch. The Vet worked on him for a week with little success. I immediately returned to Princeton finding an unhappy and miserable pooch. I tried everything to help him walk with no success. He couldn't even wag his tail. We cried together! I had him peacefully euthanized.

Upon returning to school, I cried for days. Edith Bailey, a classmate of mine, came into my room. "Cecil, I'm sorry about Pooh. How can I help?" she asked.

"No one can do anything. I've lost my best friend. Why Mother let him go down those steps is beyond me. Because Mike works a second job at night and doesn't get home until around 9:30, Mother sleeps late in the mornings. Pooh probably had to release himself and rushed down the stairs. Oh, I'm so upset with her," I answered, tears running down my face.

"Come on. Let's go to dinner. Food will make you feel better," Edith assured me. She was right. I hadn't eaten for days.

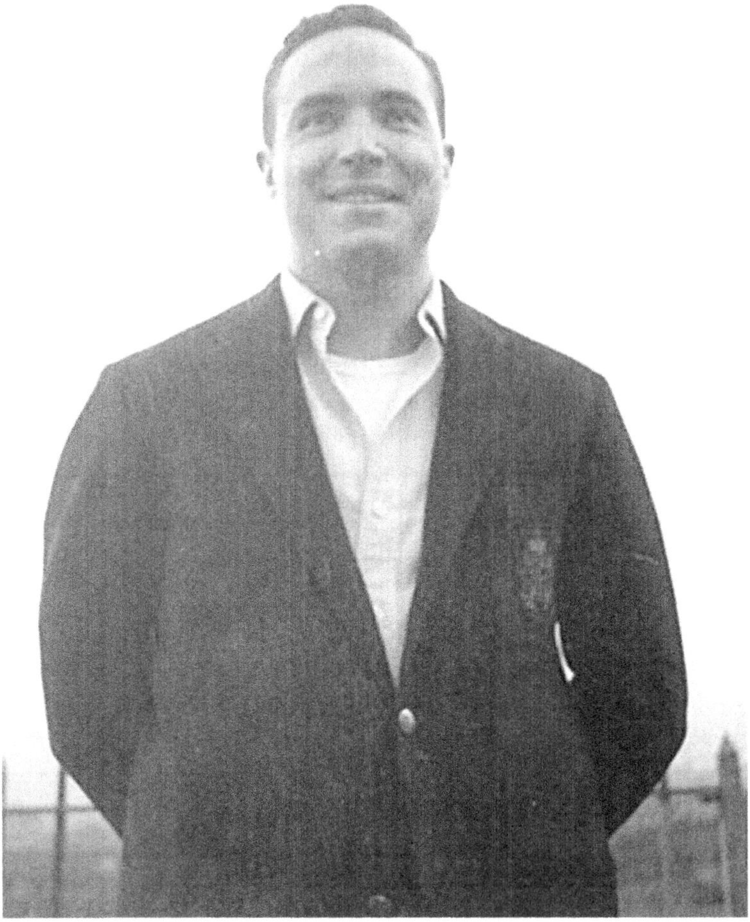

Peter in third year at Columbia Law School, 1959

# How We Met

Much to my surprise, after dinner the next night, and after Pooh's passing on Tuesday, February 11th, the phone rang down the hall from my room at St. Luke's. I had just stepped out of the shower.

"Ceci, it's for you," someone shouted.

"I'm coming," I shouted back. Who would be calling me, I wondered, and picked up the phone's receiver. "Hello?"

"Cecil (as my classmate, Edith Bailey, called me), this is Alan," he said.

"Hey," I responded adjusting my towel.

"Edith is here. Can you join us tonight?" he asked. "I'd like you to meet my roommate, Peter Hitchcock."

"I'd love to but not tonight. I've just taken a shower and need to curl my hair," I said. "I should study also."

"Please," Alan begged. "It won't be a late night."

"I'm sorry Alan . . . absolutely not, but I'll take a rain check!" I said.

"Well O.K. . . . another time," Alan sighed and hung up the phone.

The next afternoon on Wednesday, February 12, 1959 (a date we always celebrated), Peter called. He asked to meet me that night. We agreed to meet in St. Luke's lobby.

A charming Peter stood out in the crowd. We immediately came in eye contact. "Ceci?" Peter asked. "Yes," I responded. We laughed. What an adorable, handsome guy. He was dressed in khaki pants and a navy blue wool jacket with its gold and maroon Princeton Charter Club, crested chest pocket. A bit of his undershirt appeared under his white oxford, a fashion he learned while in the Navy in England when out of uniform. How preppy he was - about 5'10" with dark brown wavy hair, sparkling hazel eyes, and a gorgeous smile. There was something about him that made my heart pound. Later, he told me he found me quite special.

"Do you mind walking five blocks?" he asked as he opened the lobby door to the outside.

"No. . .no! I love walking," I responded smiling. "In this crowded and busy City, it's a fast way to get to your destination because of the horrific traffic.

"You're right! By the way, I'm sorry about Pooh," he said with such compassion. "I hope tonight will bring some cheer."

"He was a great dog. He meant a lot to me," I sighed, trying to be upbeat.

We hit it off immediately during our walk from 114th to 119th Street and Riverside Drive to his apartment which was very close to Columbia University.

We had so much in common. We talked about Exeter, which he loved, and Princeton. Most of my male family members went to the University. Much to my surprise, Peter's date, along with his roommate, Keith McLean's date, almost stayed at our house on Cleveland Lane. My Mother, Mrs. Ginny Kohlsaat, had decided to rent a room, which was hard to come by in town. The boys decided against it because the walk was too far from campus. My sister, Starr, was recently married to Dunham Wilson, Class of 1950 . . . probably that was Starr's room Mother wanted to rent.

"I have a funny story," I said chuckling. "Dunham and his roommate stole the clapper from Princeton's Nassau Hall bell. They waited until dark one night and went to the back wing of the building, where the 2nd Continental Congress once met. Finding a ladder, left by a window washer, they climbed up to the cupola. Dunham saw the Proctor and hid under the bell. The Proctor periodically checked the bell by pulling the cord which in turn hit Dunham on the head (a bump he had for the rest of his life according to my sister); however, the two boys were able to steal the clapper, which they hid in the fireplace in the dorm room. The University had told the students, that if they could hide the clapper for three days, they could keep it. Dunham had it sawed in half." To this day, Starr has it hanging on her living room wall!" Peter and I burst out laughing.

Another surprise was that Peter's Aunt Deborah, sister of his father, went to St. Mary's, Class of 1919.

"How about that!" exclaimed Peter with a warm grin. "Seems we have a lot in common."

"It's certainly a small world, isn't it," I said. We couldn't get over the fact that we both were in Princeton at the same time and never met. I dated many students and had gone club hopping frequently at Charter Club, Peter's Club.

The boy's first floor flat was in a college-rented building. It was small, but cozy, with two bedrooms, bath, and a sizeable living room with an island and a kitchen at one end.

Edith and I had become good friends. She was such a good-natured person, always making people laugh. She did, however, have a bad habit of twirling and twisting strands of her long brown curly hair no matter where she was. As for Alan, I had heard so much about him from her. I was anxious to meet him. The two met through a friend of Edie's. Alan wanted to give her an engagement ring but she held off . . . said she wasn't ready. Just like Peter, Alan was quite a jokester, at that, and extremely good-looking.

We all cracked up that evening. Edie and I learned all about Bessy, the cleaning lady. "She'd do a great job of cleaning," said Peter chuckling. "She'd do anything for us…changing beds, scrubbing the kitchen and bath, even washing clothes. Nevertheless, late one afternoon after Bessy had left the apartment, we returned from class." Peter stopped. He and Alan roared with laughter.

"What happened?" I begged them laughing.

"She had taken a nip!" answered Alan, trying to restrain himself. He pointed to the table in the corner. "We found those framed pictures upside down."

"And the empty whiskey bottle was hidden in the bottom of the garbage pail," Peter remarked.

"So that's why the liquor is in the closet," giggled Edith.

"Uh huh!" Peter chortled, "Under lock and key." I looked at my watch. "Gosh it's getting late," I said. "Do you mind walking me back? I hate to interrupt. Tonight's been fun."

"Not at all," Peter answered as he got up from the armchair.

We said "goodnight" to Edie and Alan and left the apartment. Edie probably would spend the night. On the way to St. Luke's Peter asked, "Have you made plans for Friday night?"

"I was going to Princeton, but I can always do that some other weekend," I responded. "Isn't Friday Valentine's Day?" I was surprised that he asked me!

"Yes, a perfect time to see you again. How about dinner?" Peter beamed, his eyes sparkling. "I enjoyed tonight."

"I'd love that," I said enthusiastically. "I haven't laughed that hard for months!"

Peter opened the lobby door and said with a broad grin, "I'll pick you up at six pm. Have a good night."

"You too," I answered back. "Thanks again." I was excited that he wanted to see me again. It seemed strange, but I think we both wanted to kiss each other.

On Valentine's evening Peter gave me a red rose and served a delicious lamb chop dinner. Afterwards, I presented him with a box of chocolate creams which we enjoyed while cleaning up the kitchen. What a great night. He wanted to kiss me goodnight, but I said it was too soon. "Ooh!" he sighed. "Maybe next time!"

From the time we met we became inseparable. I found Peter to be lots of fun as he had a dry wit. He was a gentleman, a history buff, bright, caring and sexy. Peter said he found me beautiful, fun, an excellent cook, and extremely prim and proper. I wanted our relationship to become special. It was awhile before we became intimate.

We both melted into each other's arms when we did. That is when "Yes please" was created. You will see us using these words throughout conversations in this book…it was a wonderful way of communicating and quite therapeutic.

We frequently prepared dinners at the apartment, sometimes with Edie and Alan. The boys were hysterical together always kidding each other. Peter was famous for Poule a la Hitchcock, baked chicken doused with brandy. I'll never forget opening the refrigerator door once and finding a Mason jar full of green liquid with white foam on top. "What is that?" I asked. "Juices from steamed vegetables," he answered back.

"A nice idea but I'll let you drink that!" I said. "It's a little aged." We both laughed. I gave him a hug as I admired the flamed chicken. It was a perfect dinner, though in the future he left the cooking up to me!

*****

In the spring of 1959, both of us prepared for finals.

Peter commented, "I won't be able to see you or talk on the phone for six weeks. Alan and I will be taking the Bar Review."

"Don't forget me," I joked. "Why don't we make use of the United States Postal Service? We can write each other (this began our writing love letters to one another).

"What a good idea!" he said smiling. "Wish we didn't have to cram but passing the New York State Bar is first priority."

"Absolutely," I agreed.

Peter kissed me on the lips. "I must go as I have classes this afternoon," I whispered and kissed him back. I proceeded to walk down the many, many steps of Columbia. When I hit the bottom I turned around. Peter waved, as I did, and I began my way back to St. Luke's. I hated to go, but I reminded myself that I, too, would be busy with finals.

# Our Courtship

I took my finals, and it would be months before Peter would hear the results of the Bar. We exchanged letters back and forth. I even sent witty and raunchy cards. In one letter, since Peter was a fan of Rupert Brooke, the poet, I pretended to be Ruperta Brooke from the Old Country. . . England. Peter's response to one of my cards:

> June 30, 1959
> "From: P. Hitchcock, Esq.
> Bickering Commons
> Niggling
> Surly
>
> Dear Ceci:
>
> Many thanks for the card, O Ruperta. I really enjoyed it. The literary touch becomes you, as so many other things, of course.
>
> Things continue grim, as far as the bar goes. What with the pressure and the oppressive heat, Alan and I have a full-time job trying to keep our heads, and remain civil to one another. You are lucky to be spared such churls as we are at present.
>
> To add to the shortage of time, my Aunt died Sunday necessitating another trip to Bronxville. (I don't mean that to appear heartless as it sounds though).
>
> What thoughts have you had about jobs, apartments, etc.? New York is a City which definitely is improved when you're around (I do miss you, old girl, actually believe it or not). At any rate, I could certainly use a morale-boosting letter from you, or else from that girl, Ruperta, who reminds me so much of the Old Country.
>
> I'd better sign off, before I drift happily off into Inanity that handmaiden of Lethe, Bacchus, and Morpheus . . . Due to the shortage of humdrum, however, I may soon start chasing Inanity in a more wholehearted manner.
>
> Lots of Love
> Peter"

Edith and I decided in June 1959 to drop out of St. Luke's much to the dismay of our parents. I had been out of school two years working as an

Executive Secretary for D. Van Nostrand Co. in Princeton. I wanted an apartment and a job.

Mike Morgan, my stepfather, called Peter begging him to get me to change my mind; thus, Peter called, "Ceci, Mike just called me. He's upset that you're leaving St. Luke's." "I'm not surprised but wish he hadn't bothered you. I'll call mother. She'll understand just like you do," I said. "I really want to leave."

After the Bar and graduation in the top quarter of his class, earning his Juris Doctor, Peter moved to Greenwich Village. The lovely garden apartment was passed on to him by Ned Boody, who had gotten married to Mary and offered the apartment. In the summer of 1958, Peter had worked for the law firm of Patterson, Belknap, Webb, and Tyler in the City. In the summer of 1959, he joined Allied Chemical Corporation on Rector Street in lower Manhattan, deciding to go into Corporate Law instead of joining a law firm. It was a big decision. In the meantime, Alan joined the law firm of Davis, Polk and Wardwell.

That summer I lived in Princeton, interviewing in the City. I then accepted a job working for J. J. James, M. D., a neurologist, and lived at the Phoebe Warren Women's' Hotel. I became friends with Kellie Moore, settling in an apartment in Midtown. I found that I was spending more time with Peter than at the apartment. I eventually moved to Jane Street in the Village and accepted a job at New York University as Executive Secretary to Charles E. Cox, retired Chairman of the Kennecott Copper Corporation, New York City, for the "75 Million Capital Fund for Leadership and Service" Campaign. I loved the work, but after a year it was discontinued. I transferred to NYU's Student Credit and Loan Department in charge of scholarships and loans, which I enjoyed, as I was working directly with students.

Ironically, Peter and I lived right down the street from each other. The only drawback was that I could never walk alone at night on poorly lit Jane Street since there were large, vacant warehouses (now apartments) across the street from my building. We were together mostly on weekends, and sometimes midweek in the evenings, enjoying Off-Broadway and Broadway shows and trying different restaurants and cuisines. Peter loved to collect ticket stubs and Playbills. Our favorite restaurants were "Patty's Clam House" at Penn Station, for we adored oysters, and "The Little Place", an Italian restaurant on 4th Street and 8th Avenue in the Village. Not only was the food excellent but we were serenaded by Jimmy, the owner. He would sing operatic arias throughout the evening reaching with great depth to everyone present. Peter always ordered the Seafood Diavolo: clams, mussels, shrimp, calamari, and scallops with homemade marinara over linguine. I adored Eggplant Parmesan!

Other times we found ourselves enjoying "The Little Italian Deli" on the corner of Jane Street. The owner would always have heated firewood warmed by a portable heater, which Peter used in his apartment fireplace. He also was a great butcher, and his meats were outstanding. We would rotate having dinner one night at his place and the other at my apartment, work permitting.

One Wednesday evening in October 1959, I was reading The New York Times in my apartment. I always picked up the paper on my way home from work, as we were told that the results of the Bar would come out in it. I happened to come across the announcement of the New York State Bar – 930 of 1,938 passed. I found Peter's and Alan's names, and immediately called Peter at work. "Congratulations...I knew you could do it!" I said. "How about that!" exclaimed Peter. "To think we had to hear through The Times." "YEAH!" I cried out. "I'm certainly proud of you. Be sure to call Alan."

*****

Looking back to when we first met, we had a few unforgettable times. We had a memorable weekend at the Hitchcock's seasonal, partially winterized home, "Thurtilperk Hill," in New Boston, Massachusetts in the Berkshires. It was built in 1923 for Peter's grandfather, the late Charles Joseph Tilden, a Professor of Engineering at Harvard. He met the late Ned Thurston, Professor of Engineering at Yale, and they became friends. Ned gave Charles the land.

Peter's mother insisted that we have a chaperone for appearance sake; thus, we invited Edie and Alan! We drove up old Route 22 in New York in the little, black four-door Vauxhall. Peter turned onto Route 7 in Connecticut, where we stopped off for dinner at The White Hart Inn in Salisbury. The Inn had been established as a small town tavern in 1806. Over the years, it was renovated, becoming a large overnight Inn with picture perfect charm.

We always had fun with Edith and Alan. It was an hilarious evening what with all the jokes and storytelling. The filet mignons were excellent, and the boys enjoyed the martinis, for which the Inn was famous.

"Who's going to finish the drive up to New Boston?" I asked. "Edie can't drive." The boys looked at me. "You are!" Alan answered back.

"I am, am I? I haven't driven a stick shift car for quite a while...well...OK!" I sighed. "I'll try."

"Good," Peter laughed, handing me the car keys

I started the car . . . off we went, but I had forgotten to put my foot on the clutch. The car jerked back and forth straight across the parking lot.

"Beads...beads," Alan shouted. "You're supposed to put your foot on the clutch and accelerate, letting the clutch out gradually!"

"Now you stop that," I snapped back, trying not to laugh. "I know what I'm doing! Don't worry. I'll get you to New Boston."

"Cecil can do it," Edith assured the laughing boys. She and I looked at each other and began to laugh so hard tears poured down our faces.

We reached New Boston, driving through back roads with our headlights to light the way. Soon I found myself driving up a steep, winding road over three meadows (the old Right-of-Way) surrounded by horses, and crossing a creosoted bridge which led to the house.

"Wow!" I exclaimed as I stopped the car. "What a haven this is Peter. I can't wait to see everything in the daylight."

"Sweet-Love, leave the headlights on so I can unlock the kitchen door. We have no electricity," he said as he leaned over and kissed me on the cheek. "Yes please!" I said handing him the car keys. Peter soon returned with flashlights. As we got out of the car there was a loud "hoot…hooting" high up in a pine tree, probably a Barred Owl. I "hooted" back causing the small bird to flail its wings and fly off. We laughed.

Peter told Alan to light the gas refrigerator to house the food we had brought up from the City. That was not an easy task as Alan found out. He had to lie down on the floor, strike a match, yet hold the gas button down to light the pilot. Meanwhile, Peter lit several kerosene lamps for Edie and me, and headed out to the pump house to start the gas pump for water, which would be stored in a large tank in the attic of the house.

In the meantime, Edie and I wandered from the small quaint kitchen into a large L-shaped dining/living room with an enormous Fieldstone fireplace. There was a long hall leading to three bedrooms and a bath. Throughout the house the walls were of oak paneling with wide board floors. Beautiful antiques decorated the entire house. To make the beds, we found linens in a mahogany bureau in one bedroom, and wool blankets in an over-sized steamer trunk in another bedroom.

All chores accomplished, we were tired and turned in for the night. Peter and I snuggled and drifted happily off into the world of Inanity. The next day the weather was warm and picture perfect. Alan, a talented fisherman, borrowed the car and went to the Clam River to catch trout for dinner. Edith relaxed in an Adirondack chair that faced Bear Mountain in the distance. She was reading a book from the Hitchcock's library. Meanwhile, Peter busied himself around the property organizing the barn and checking on the guest cottage and pump house.

As for me, I volunteered to brush aluminum paint behind the gas tanks to protect the yellow stained wall outside the kitchen. Peter was overjoyed. "My parents will so appreciate your doing this," he commented.

*****

For dinner we enjoyed Alan's fresh water trout – quite a treat! We ate, not by candlelight, but by light from two gas mantels above the dining room table. The four of us laughed over a glass of wine and hearing about hilarious experiences Alan and Peter had had together or in their schools. Alan had gone to Yale University, Class of 1953, a great rival of Princeton. Both were competitive in sports, especially the Yale-Princeton football games. From 1949 to 1951, the Princeton Tigers had the renowned Dick Kazmaier, a winner of the Heisman Trophy, on their team. I too enjoyed all his exciting games but never once bumped into Peter.

Later that night Peter and I had our first fight. Edith and Alan had gone to bed. Peter was sitting in the wicker rocking chair in front of the fire he had built in the enormous Fieldstone fireplace. I sat down on his lap. He kissed me on the cheek. "Ah! Yes please," I sighed giving him a hug.

"I love this place. I love everything about it, even the antique furniture, especially the spinning wheel and the mahogany cradle," I continued. "And your fire is absolutely perfect and beautiful."

Much to my surprise, Peter interrupted. "What kind of reception do you want?" Bewildered, I gave his question a great deal of thought. How do I answer I wondered? "I'd like a small reception in Princeton, in our 1800 colonial house with its "Gone with the Wind" staircase," I said. It was a six bedroom Clapboard Stedman house, as were the houses around us on Mercer and Alexander Streets and in the community. Mike's father lived there in 1906.

"No," Peter declared. "It has to be big. My parents will probably invite many friends from Bronxville, New York, and my father's clients. They'd have to travel to Princeton. Someone would have to feed them."

"Your parents," I answered back. "We could have the rehearsal dinner that Friday night."

"I'm not sure," he responded. "The reception can't be small." Before I could say another word, I heard, "I was going to marry Stacey."

"Well, what makes you think that Phillip Morehouse is out of the picture?" I asked, trying to make him jealous. "He took me to dinner to The Tavern on the Green in Central Park just last week. He also calls me frequently from South Carolina." Peter gave me a strange look. He was shocked! I was getting madder by the minute. "Why did you want to talk about a reception? Go marry Stacey," I cried out, as I got down from his lap and stormed off to bed. I was crushed.

The next morning, Peter turned over in bed and stroked my blond hair. He kissed me on the forehead, my back turned away from him. "I'm sorry for last night," he whispered in my ear. "I'm not going to marry Stacey." I was so moved and glad.

"I'm sorry, too," I said turning over. "But I didn't enjoy our fighting."

"I know...by the way, you're beautiful when you get mad," he commented smiling. "Do you love Phillip?"

"No," I answered.

"Then I'd like to show you just how much you mean to me...come here," he said and kissed me on the lips.

"I'd liked that...Yes please!" I answered back, stroking his thick brown hair, as I stared into his laughing eyes. We then entered the world of Inanity, my Sweet-Love and I.

Late that morning, after a banana-walnut muffin and a cup of coffee, Peter and Alan decided to explore the area on foot, while Edie and I prepared lunch, which would take some time to make. While I fixed a tossed spring salad with sliced strawberries and roasted pecans, Edie took care of the chicken. She soaked a large cast iron pot with liquid detergent and ammonia. The pot was meant to hang on a swinging bracket over the fire in the Fieldstone fireplace.

"That!" I said pointing to the pot. "Are you sure that is a good way to clean it?"

"Don't worry Cecil. I'll take care of it," she assured me. She began scrubbing the pot, finally rinsing it over and over again.

"Let the pot soak with water until we're ready," I suggested. "Just be sure or we'll all get sick!"

I made an olive oil and balsamic dressing, and then built a large Girl Scout's fire in the fireplace. Edith added the vegetable oil to the empty pot and began to fry the cut-up chicken.

"Boy, does that smell good!" Peter remarked, as he and Alan walked into the house. It did, but I still had my doubts and hoped the chicken wouldn't make us sick; otherwise, our lunch was a great success.

"Edith, you did a good job," I said smiling.

Late that afternoon we tidied up the house, turned off the gas/water pump and refrigerator, and headed back to the City. This time Peter drove.

"Everyone feeling OK?" I asked, my stomach beginning to churn! "A little queasy," was the reply. We made it back to the City without any mishaps, thank goodness.

A wonderful time was had by all, but we agreed we'd never cook chicken in that pot again.

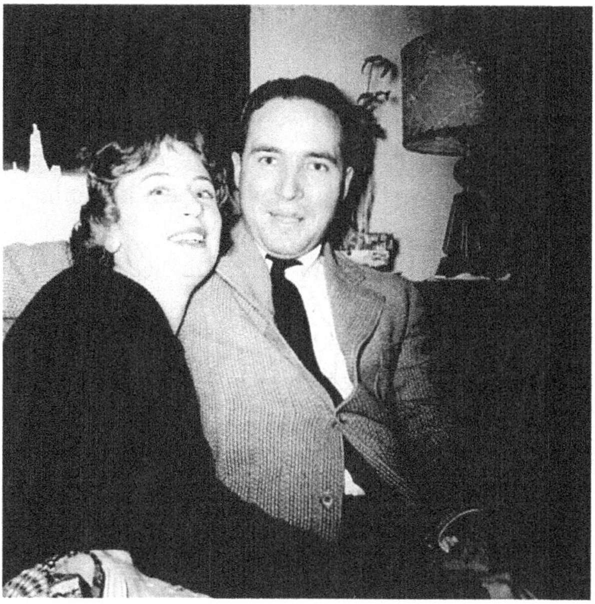

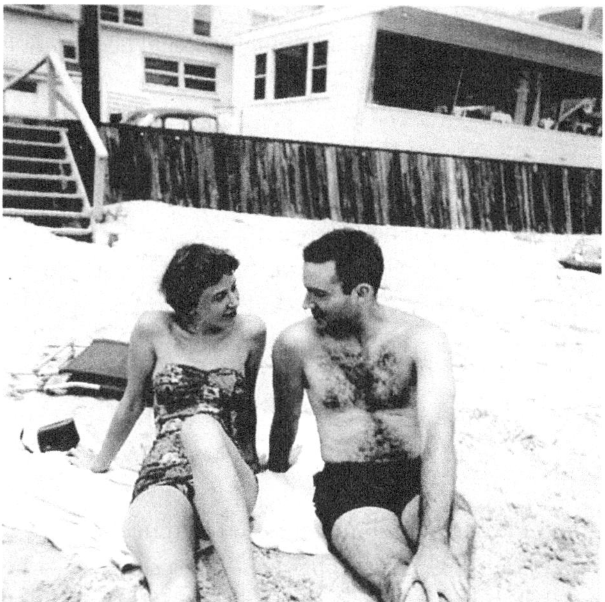

## Meeting My Parents

I invited Peter in August to meet my parents at their rented house in Stone Harbor in southern New Jersey. Peter drove down early Saturday morning after picking up the Vauxhall in Bronxville, the night before.

Mother greeted him at the front door just as I was coming down the stairs from the second floor. I had been making his bed.

"Hi, Peter," she said in such a warm way. "I'm glad to meet you finally. Ceci has told us all about you. Please come in."

"I hope it was good," Peter laughed.

"Hey," I said smiling. I'm happy to see you." We wanted to kiss but Mike got up from his crossword puzzle table.

"So nice to meet you, Mike," greeted Peter happily. "We've talked on the phone recently about Ceci leaving St. Luke's."

"Greetings," Mike responded shaking hands. "We did indeed. How was your trip?"

"There was a bit of traffic on the Garden State Parkway but, all in all, it wasn't too bad."

"I've just made lunch...I hope you're hungry!" I said. "Come into the kitchen. Mike just carved the ham, while I made potato salad. I thought we could have ham sandwiches. Mother bought some beautiful, luscious Jersey tomatoes which we can have...a real treat."

"Sounds good to me, Sweet-Love," Peter said as he put his suitcase at the bottom of the stairway. Mother walked into the kitchen with us.

"Stone Harbor certainly is a lovely town. Thank you for inviting me, Ginny," Peter remarked taking a bite of his sandwich.

"We come here every August. We've been doing it for nine years," she answered. "You'll love the beach. It shouldn't be too crowded. Kathy and Dick Zundal, good friends of ours, arrive tomorrow. Please excuse me as I have a few things to do."

"Your parents certainly are hospitable and nice. Just like you, Sweet-Love," beamed Peter as he leaned over the table and kissed me.

"Ah, Yes please," I said. "I'm so glad to see you. I think you're pretty wonderful but don't let that build up your ego too much!"

"Never...never," Peter kidded. "That could never happen. I'm so glad to see you, too. I've missed you."

*****

After cleaning up the kitchen, I showed Peter his room. It was next to mine. We changed into our bathing suits. Holding hands, we then headed to the beach which was two blocks from the house...so happy to be together. When we reached the bulkhead I kissed Peter on the cheek. "I just felt like doing that," I laughed. Peter squeezed my hand.

"Your mother was right. It isn't crowded," he remarked walking down the steps to the beach. We enjoyed the warm sand under our feet. The sun beat down upon us. It felt good, as I spread a blanket near the water's edge.

"Sweetheart, now you can relax, away from busy city life," I commented smiling as we sat down.

"And I can't wait for you to move into the City. That will be nice," he responded with such a beautiful smile on his face.

"I hope to get there soon. I'm certainly working hard to find a job!" I answered back. "Why are you looking at me?"

"I'm just admiring you . . . you're beautiful . . . shiny blond hair and a dark tan . . . very sexy," he replied, kissing me on the lips.

"You're pretty handsome yourself . . . irresistible, I might add," I said.

"Ah! I like that," he said putting his hands behind his head. He had a loving, but smug, look on his face.

"Now don't let your ego get to you!" I commented. We laughed.

*****

That night Mother and Mike treated us to dinner at Hahn's Restaurant on the Island. It was crowded and very noisy. I'm glad Mike made reservations as there was quite a waiting line. We were seated immediately. We ordered swordfish...so tender and delicious, a favorite of ours. We also enjoyed the notorious Hahn's snapper soup.

When we finished dinner Mike asked, "How about a game of shuffleboard?"

"Sounds good to me," Peter answered back. Mother and Mike won, of course.

Peter and I thanked my parents and walked the two blocks to the house. The half-moon shined down upon us, the sky dotted with shimmering stars. We stopped and kissed just before going into the house. Words are so inadequate as to how we felt! I think we were falling in love.

Mother and Mike were still up, sitting out on the porch. "Ginny, do you remember when you were renting a room at 11 Cleveland Lane in Princeton in 1950? You were Ginny Kohlsaat then?" Peter asked. "My roommate, Keith McLean, and I had called asking you to put up our dates. We decided against it because the walk was too far from campus."

"You have a good memory," Mother responded. "I do remember. Mike and I were married that September. We moved to Prospect Avenue soon after right next to the baseball field. The Princeton clubs were right up the road from us. We were there two years before we bought 36 Mercer Street."

"Quite a coincidence," I commented. "Much less a small world. To think we two were living in Princeton and never met! We should head up to bed so we can get up early and enjoy the beach tomorrow. I'll be going back with Peter to the City for two interviews I have Monday."

*****

The next morning Mike, being an early riser, went to The Bakery at the end of the Island next to Avalon to buy sticky buns…a real treat on Sunday mornings. He would then return to the house to scramble eggs and cook sausages for a delicious breakfast. There would be enough for the Zundals when they arrive.

"Those sticky buns are scrumptious!" said Peter.

"The next time we come back, they will be our treat," I commented. "Thank you so much, Mike. Peter will have to taste your fried eggplant sometime!"

*****

After breakfast I washed the dishes and suggested that we not go to the beach but head on back to the City.

"Good idea!" Peter exclaimed. "Besides the sky is overcast and not a beach day."

"Are you sure?" I asked. "There will be traffic."

"Absolutely, Sweet-Love," he answered smiling. We packed our suitcases and thanked Mother and Mike, who walked us to the front door. "I'll keep in touch with you," I said and kissed Mother on the cheek. As we were about to get into the Vauxhall, the Zundals pulled up in front of the house.

"Hi Kathy," I greeted her as she got out of the car. I gave her a kiss on the cheek. "I'd like you to meet Peter."

"So nice to meet you," Peter said happily. "And you must be Dick?" They shook hands.

"Mother and Mike are on the porch," I said. "We're on our way back to the City."

"It's wonderful seeing you," Kathy shouted as she climbed the steps to the house.

"Have a good trip," Dick said.

*****

Peter and I did have a fairly good trip back. We were glad we left when we did as getting into the City was hectic. Traffic was backed up, and finding a parking space outside Peter's apartment was even harder.

We were happy to be alone. We then went to "The Little Place" for dinner, and I spent the night.

"Alone at last," Peter beamed. "You know what I want to do?"

"Do you really want me to answer that?" I kidded.

"No, Sweet-Love," he said taking my hand and leading me into the bedroom. We melted into each other's arms and entered into the world of Inanity.

*****

The next morning Peter slipped out of bed and made coffee before getting ready for work.

"My interview isn't until ten am," I commented. "Would you like a fried egg and toast?"

"I'd love it, Sweet-Love," Peter shouted from the bathroom. He was shaving. I laughed. I quickly got dressed and prepared the breakfast.

"How do you want your egg?" I shouted from the kitchen.

"Sunny-side up," he answered back from the bedroom. He soon came into the dining room and sat down. "Thanks so much," he said gulping down the food hurriedly. "Never have I known anyone as sweet as you!"

"You're pretty sweet yourself. I enjoyed last night," I answered laughing. "You go on ... I'll clean up. I'll be leaving shortly for the interviews in Midtown."

"Thanks again," he said reaching into his pocket. "Here's the key to the apartment." He kissed me on the lips and opened the front door. "I'll call you tonight...bye." I was so proud of him. He looked so handsome in his three-piece dark gray suit.

*****

Much to my surprise, J. J. James, M. D., the neurologist, wanted to hire me on the spot. I wasn't sure because of the low salary. I'd let him know. The other job opportunity was filled. I then visited the Phoebe Warren Womens' Hotel, where I planned to live after I found a job and looked for an apartment. Soon after I took the next train from Penn Station to Princeton, for I had decided to work through an agency.

*****

The end of the month, on Labor Day weekend, I invited Peter, Edie, and Alan to Stone Harbor for Saturday and Sunday. My parents had guests; thus, the boys made reservations at a Cape May motel.

Upon their arrival we went to the house, said "hello" to everyone, changed into bathing suits, and headed for the beach.

Edie and Alan decided to take a walk to the Inlet. As usual, the beach was crowded but we didn't care. The tide was going out with little undertow, so we were able to push our way out beyond the waves that crashed against the beach. The salty water was warm, the breeze refreshing as the sun beat down upon us.

"Look…out in the distance," I said to Peter pointing as I put my head on his shoulder. "Sweet-Love," he said nudging me. Against the horizon there were several fishing boats surrounded by seagulls. Close by, a pod of playful dolphins danced in a row, vaulting up and down in the calm sea. Over by the Inlet, we could see Edie and Alan watching seagulls crack mussels by dropping them on the rocky bank. The whole scene had picture-perfect charm.

Peter and I left the water and walked up to the bulkhead where we had left our belongings. I spread a blanket on the sand as we lay down, the sand crunching underneath us. In those days (the 50's) we never, or rarely, wore sunglasses, much less used sunscreen. If anything, we used baby oil with a drop of Iodine to get a tan!

Edie and Alan soon joined us from their walk bringing back quite a collection of seashells, which they had put in Alan's Yale cap. Edie wanted to fill a glass lamp base with shells.

The four of us managed to put our clothes on over our dry bathing suits and head to Hahn's Restaurant for dinner. The surf and turf was delicious as was the snapper soup. After dinner, Peter and I challenged Alan and Edie to shuffleboard. We won, much to Alan's chagrin. Soon after, we reached the run-down motel in Cape May. Our room was no bigger than 10 feet by 12 feet with a double bed, a torn overstuffed chair, and a bathroom that truly needed renovating. The smell of mildew and dead clams from low tide permeated the room. But we didn't care. We had clean sheets. That's all that mattered. We just wanted to be together.

The next morning, after a hearty breakfast at a Cape May diner, I said "goodbye" to Edie and Alan, and kissed Peter. I hated to see them go but they had to catch the Cape May Ferry to the inland. I was to stay behind to help my parents close up the house and return to Princeton on Labor Day.

*****

"The Princeton Club of New York
Park Avenue and 39th Street
New York 16, New York

August 26, 1959

Dear Ceci,

Sorry I didn't get a chance to write to you Sunday. I felt a letter coming on, but got to Bronxville so late that fatigue had dulled all muses. We had a pleasant trip, but had to wait 45 minutes for the ferry – it's a good idea going down, but less advantageous coming back.

I'm working at the Bar Association Library this evening, dropped over here for dinner, and suddenly felt a letter coming on.

Saturday I'll probably do some lawyering (if it rains) or else catch up on the back gardening. Sunday the boat ride, then back to the usual.

Let me know how your plans progress, please.

This last weekend was an extremely happy one, a tribute to your organizational talent as well as your niceness to be around.

Missing you,

Lots of love,

Peter"

"Hi, my Darling,August 25, 1959

Ah! Old Ruperta is far into Inanity in a state of trance due to the powers of Lethe, enticed by the pleasures of Bacchus, and subdued by the charm of Morpheus. Yes, twas a perfect weekend for sure. I must admit I felt somewhat depressed and lonely after you left- a few tears fell, without being obvious, as you three got into the car and pulled away from the house. I hated to see you leave and as a cure I managed to sleep for several hours.

There have been no repercussions as to the motel here. The only remark made was by Mike. "I'm sure the boys must be broke after taking you and Edie out for so many meals! You should have gotten them to eat more here." He is so right about the money side of it. I wish there hadn't been a deadline of 11 a.m. this morning. Yes, I was somnolent, but Yes please!! Even with all the mosquitos and the smell of mildew, the room was tres wonderful and made the whole weekend completely and positively perfect. Ah, Mr. Hitchcock, I find you most wonderful and I miss you already.

May I hear from you in the next few days whether it be by letter or by phone. I know how tired you are to even think of writing after a day's work. But you are greatly missed, and oh, do I wish you were here now!

Lots of Love,

Ruperta"

"Weekapaug Inn
Weekapaug, R.I.

Dear Ceci:

All is well here, the R.I. sunning and swimming here have been good, although I'm sure I won't be able to match the black tan which you doubtless have acquired by now.

We're leaving here Thursday morning. I'll call you that evening. At present there appear to be no hitches in weekend plans, particularly since I can plead sanctity of vacations, etc. If all is still the same at your end, I would expect to head down Friday night or early Saturday morning, bringing you back Sunday night or Monday morning.

Miss you,
Lots of love,
Peter"

August 29, 1959
"Cecily Gates Kohlsaat
36 Mercer Street
Princeton, New Jersey

Dearest Peter:

I feel so happy and bubbling over – seems I should be down in the dumps since having little success with jobs this afternoon, but Ah, I'm not! Guess I'm accustomed to pot luck when it comes to job hunting, but your letter was a morale booster. Was so happy to hear from you – and as you would say, I felt a letter coming on. I miss you, and also would like to let you know of my plans for next week.

I must say though, it was a coincident receiving your letter this morning; that is, I dreamed I had received one from you – then in the dream you, Edie, and Alan suddenly pulled up in front of the house in P-town. We proceeded to drive to Stone Harbor taking a long, unknown way! Strangely enough the hills were covered with snow yet it wasn't cold for the top was down on the car. Sound familiar? Anyway, we arrived at the motel, the rooms unlocked (not by Ulrich though) and of course, I woke up.

I called the Agency this afternoon whereby I received several opportunities besides the ones I had. Two look very promising.

Tuesday around nine am I will head into the City to see the Agency upon their request, as there are "many vacancies" open. I shall try my darndest for I would like to start work, on the 8$^{th}$. Would there be a possibility of seeing you? Suppose I call you on Monday night, if that is o.k.? Perhaps we can get together sometime during next week; that is, if you haven't made plans or have to work in the wee hours of the night.

I miss you, Darling, and I hope we can get together very soon.

Lots of love,

Ceci

P.S. I found out where Hahn's Restaurant gets its snapper soup! Marty Hahn, the son, is getting the address for me – I know it is Adam's Canning Co., Philadelphia though."

After having several more interviews and talking to Peter and my parents, I decided to work for J. J. James, M. D. I would start on September 8$^{th}$ but would move into the Phoebe Warren Womens' Hotel after Labor Day.

During that fall on Saturdays, Peter and I would drive down in the Vauxhall to Princeton to tailgate behind the Charter Club with friends at the University's home football games. We were lucky because Mother worked at the Athletic Club, where she presented us with 50 yard seats!

*****

Edie and Alan were married the winter of 1960. Peter was best man and I was maid of honor. I found it quite awkward walking up the aisle of the church by myself. Facing Peter was even harder, wishing I was in Edie's place; however, Peter smiled at me several times which made me feel better.

After the short ceremony there was a small reception in the parish hall. It was very nice as we were among friends. I joined Peter.

"Sweet-Love, you looked so handsome standing next to Alan. The ceremony was lovely, wasn't it?" I asked. "I did feel strange walking up the aisle by myself."

"You did well," he replied. "I like your dress, very sexy! You are certainly beautiful." I laughed. "But your haircut," he continued. "It's much too short."

"I can always grow it back. Edie wanted it this way," I said looking into his sparkling hazel eyes.

"Cecil, come join us," Edith shouted from across the room. The single girls grouped together waiting in anticipation. "Ready?" Edith asked.

"Yes," I shouted, as I handed Peter my bouquet of flowers. I found myself jumping high up in the air. Much to my amazement I had caught Edith's flowers.

Returning to Peter, I commented, "It is said that the one who catches the bridal bouquet is the next one to be married."

"How about that!" Peter said with a big smile on his face.

Someone touched me on the shoulders. I turned around. Peter decided to visit with a close friend, Baus, a classmate at Columbia Law School. "I'm Mary Vaughn," she said. She was a petite girl with long straight red hair.

"Hello," I said wondering what she wanted.

"You know, Peter and I almost became engaged," she commented.

"Really?" I snapped. "You wish!" I immediately left her and joined Peter and Baus. Later I asked Peter about Mary. "Don't believe a word she says. Yes, I did date her once," he said laughing. "She'll do and say anything to get a man. Alan dated her several times. But that's all." I felt better but wondered why she had been invited…such a strange person.

We were so happy that Edie and Alan finally got married, as Edie had broken off the engagement once and kept putting off the wedding. They moved into the red brick high-rise on 12th Street, a few doors down from Peter's brownstone.

As for me, I know Peter and I were crazy in love with each other but wouldn't admit it. That is, until I slipped up!

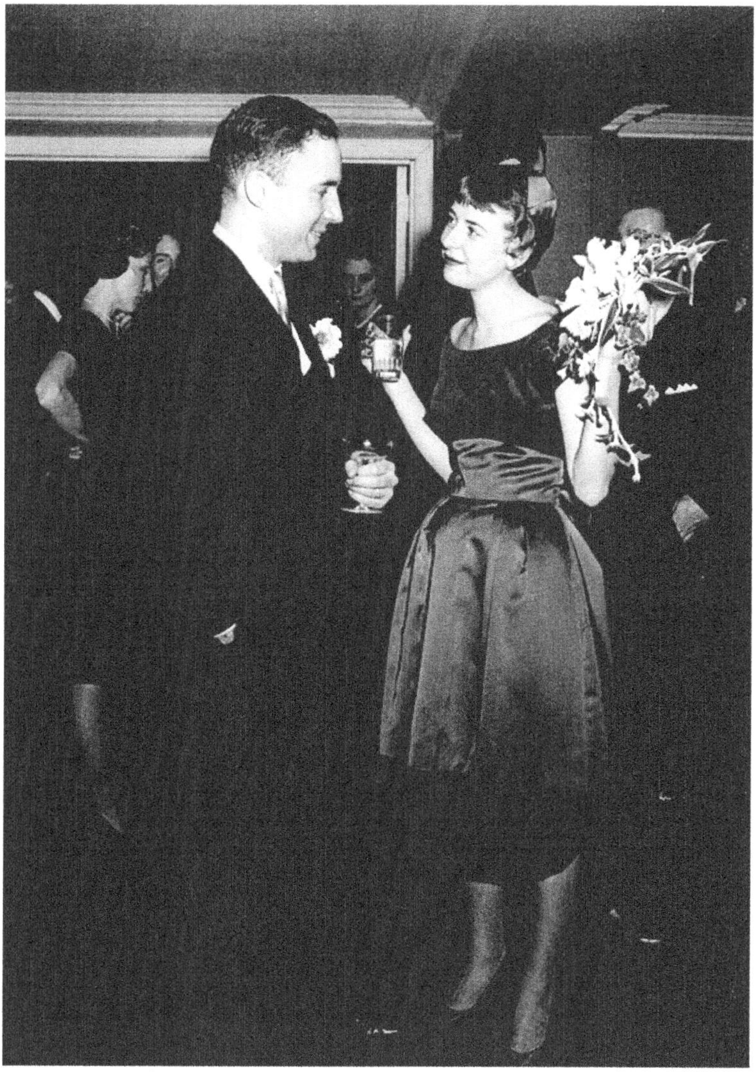

Peter and Ceci attending
Edie and Alan's Wedding, 1960

# The Slip Up

Late one Saturday evening, after having dinner in the theatre district and seeing "Fiddler on the Roof," Peter flagged a cab for me. He was to spend Sunday with his family in Bronxville. Peter handed me cash and told the cab driver to take me to 20 Jane Street.

I thanked him for a wonderful evening. We kissed and we hugged. "You know what," I whispered in his ear. "I love you."

"Uh huh!" exclaimed Peter with a warm smile on his face. He gave me a hug.

I got into the cab and panicked, realizing what I had said. For sure I've ruined our relationship, I thought. He hadn't told me that he loved me. What in the world have I done?

I waited for Peter to get to Bronxville – a very long wait! Finally, I got him on the phone. "I shouldn't have told you that I love you. It's much too soon," I said nervously.

"That's o.k., Sweet-Love. I enjoyed the evening," he reassured me. "Let's talk tomorrow. Goodnight."

"Goodnight," I responded. My mind was set at ease.

# Part Two: Wedding Belles

## The Trip to Bronxville

In late April, 1960, I was invited for the night to meet Peter's parents, Elinor and Horace Hitchcock. I was quite nervous on the train, fearing that his parents wouldn't like me; yet, I was overjoyed to be meeting them and learning a little more about Peter's home life.

When we arrived at the Bronxville Station we picked up the Vauxhall, which Peter stored in a parking garage while working in the City, and headed to Avon Road.

"Do you think your parents will like me?" I asked nervously in the car.

"Of course," he answered. "They are eager to meet you.

It was still light outside as we parked in front of the house. High up on the hill there was the most beautiful white stucco, three-story mansion trimmed in gray. Close to the front patio, a Rhododendron in full bloom with purple-pink flowers stood tall and bushy, at least two stories high.

Peter's brother, Gaylord, who is twelve years younger, ran down the steps. "Hi, Petie," he said out of breath. "I'm on my way to the high school for the operetta."

"Hi Gaylord…we'll be there," Peter answered. "I want you to meet Ceci Kohlsaat. She has come to spend the night with us."

"Hey," I said. "Peter has told me a lot about you. I hear you have a wonderful voice and love music."

"I don't know about the voice, but yes, I do love music." Gaylord laughed. "I'm always in all the operettas. Here comes my ride. See you later."

To reach the house we must have climbed 25 steps to the patio, passing the beautifully landscaped property. Elinor, Horace, and Inky, the black cat, met us at the front door.

"Finally, we meet, Ceci," Elinor said squeezing my hand. "We have talked on the phone many times, haven't we?"

"Yes, Mrs. Hitchcock," I said. "Thank you and who is this?"

"This is Inky," she responded. The cat meowed rubbing his head against my leg.

"You certainly are beautiful, Inky, and friendly, too," I said stroking him on his back.

"So nice to meet you, Mr. Hitchcock," I continued, shaking his hand. I then handed Mrs. Hitchcock a hostess present; a floral wrapped box with a pink and green bow. "I hope you will like this."

"Come and sit down," Mr. Hitchcock said, taking off my coat. "Would you like a cocktail?"

"Thank you…I'll join all of you if you're having one," I responded entering the large living room. I sat down in a lovely green, silk floral Queen Anne chair. After helping his father, Peter sat across from me in a stunning green leather chair tacked with brass nails. He winked at me and wore the greatest smile. I began to relax. Mrs. Hitchcock joined us passing cheese and crackers. We talked about everything from New Boston, to St. Mary's, Princeton, Dartmouth, where Mr. Hitchcock graduated in 1919, and City life. Peter's parents were so cordial. I felt right at home.

"Mrs. Hitchcock, may I help you with dinner?" I asked.

"No . . . no," she answered. "But we must eat soon if we're going to the operetta. "You and Peter have a seat in the dining room.

We entered a room that was decorated with light green grass wallpaper. The three-leafed mahogany dining room table, surrounded by eight exquisite chairs, rested on a plush green carpet. It was lovely.

Peter sat across from me, after helping me with my chair. He smiled at me in such a loving way. I think his parents noticed as they smiled but didn't say anything.

I admired the bone china dinner plate set in front of me and looked at the back. "I love fine china and antiques," I commented. "This is Limoges. It's beautiful." Mrs. Hitchcock seemed pleased. She served such a delicious lamb dinner followed by homemade chocolate mocha cake and vanilla ice cream.

Peter and I helped in the kitchen. I dried while Peter stacked the dishes in the butler's pantry.

After deciding to head to the Bronxville High School in two cars, Peter and I hurriedly put on our coats and drove to the school in the Vauxhall. Arriving twenty minutes early for the eight pm show enabled us to find good seats.

Gaylord, a Sophomore, did a superb job in the operetta, "Leave It to Jane," both in acting and singing. We thoroughly enjoyed the whole evening.

Arriving home, after hanging up our coats, Mr. Hitchcock announced, "Gaylord, you did well . . . now it's time for bed . . . Goodnight."

*****

We climbed the magnificent winding staircase to the second floor. Mrs. Hitchcock showed me my room. Peter handed me my suitcase and went over to the bottom of the stairs leading up to the third floor. We wanted to kiss goodnight but his mother stood between us. "Goodnight," she said. "Goodnight," we said. Peter laughed!

The next morning I awoke to a knocking sound. I put on my robe and answered the door.

"Hi, Sweetheart," I said and kissed Peter on the lips.

"Did you sleep well?" he whispered, hugging me.

"I slept like a kitten," I responded. "I love your parents."

"Good," said Peter. "They have breakfast ready. Take the stairs down to the butler's pantry."

"I'll be right down," I said. I quickly got dressed and I found the steep stairwell, Peter spoke about, halfway down the winding stairway to the first floor. "Good morning," I greeted everyone. Peter got up from his chair and helped me with my chair. "Gaylord, we so enjoyed last night. You have such talent."

"Thank you," Gaylord replied smiling.

"I hope you slept well," Mrs. Hitchcock said, as she walked around the table pouring fresh squeezed orange juice in our glasses.

"Yes . . . thank you. The bed was so comfortable," I responded. "Peter told me about your special Sunday breakfasts, Mr. Hitchcock." He smiled and began to serve from four aluminum pots stacked on top of each other, heated by Sterno. He started at the top and would put each pot on a hot tray; the first held scrambled eggs; the second toast; the third hash brown potatoes; the fourth sausage.

"What a clever idea," I said.

"Everyone enjoy!" said Mr. Hitchcock and sat down.

"Such a treat!" I exclaimed and began eating. "I love the orange juice, Mrs. Hitchcock. Thank you." Peter gave me a broad grin as Mr. Hitchcock then offered seconds.

"How did the New Boston house get its name?" I asked.

"It was created by my Father, Charles Joseph Tilden, who became friends with Ned Thurston," said Mrs. Hitchcock. He owned Snow Farm. You drove through his meadows to get to the house. I nodded "yes." "Well, 'Dampada,' as Peter called him, took the first few letters of each last name from Thurston, Tilden, and Perkins creating 'Thurtilperk.' The 'Perk' belonged to Mrs. Florence Perkins who ran a summer retreat in the house on the hill across from the Thurston barn. She is a lovely lady, who once ran The New Boston Inn.

'Dampada' named the place 'Thurtilperk Hill' which is located on Snow Mountain. Peter has been going up there since he was two years old."

"Really, I said and looked at Peter. "It's lovely and such a haven."

"Ned Thurston had a bungalow built way up behind the Perkins' house," said Mr. Hitchcock. It overlooked two tennis courts, now a stand of trees. It was Ned's retreat where he would grade school papers and play the piano."

"I'll take you up there, Ceci," Peter replied. "Unfortunately, no one has taken care of it. The walls have collapsed but the large Fieldstone fireplace and piano are still standing. Maybe we can visit Mrs. Perkins one day."

"I'd love to meet her and to see the bungalow sometime," I said. "It's too bad that it has deteriorated. I guess no one is interested in renovating it."

"You're absolutely right," said Mr. Hitchcock as he rose to his feet.

"We'll do the dishes, Daddy," Peter said. "Both you and Mommy go and relax. Thank you for a nice breakfast."

*****

Later, we took the train back to the City after thanking Peter's parents and returning the car to the garage. It was on time and would take us back to Grand Central Station. Peter helped me onto the train, which was somewhat crowded. We found seats and sat down. I put my head on his shoulder. "Thank you for a perfect weekend," I whispered. "Your parents are wonderful, just like you!"

"And so are you," Peter answered back.

*****

"Mrs. Horace G. Hitchcock
51 Avon Road
Bronxville, New York

April 24th
Dear Ceci:

Thank you for the beautiful guest towels. They are the loveliest I have had since I was first married, and I am thrilled to have them.

It was a great pleasure to have you come out for the week-end, and for Gaylord's operetta – and I hope we will see you again soon.

Sincerely,
Elinor Hitchcock

# The Proposal

In August, 1960, Peter began to work late in the evenings and some weekends. It had been almost two years since we met. I wondered if marriage was a possibility as he hadn't mentioned he loved me. Would we ever get married? I knew I loved him. Maybe competition would be a good idea!

I met with Alan and Edie one night at their apartment. Their advice was just that...competition. "When Peter wants to get married, you'll know about it," Alan said.

By coincidence, Mother called one evening to say that the Muller's son had just moved to the City. Tom didn't know anyone. "Would I like to meet him?" she asked. "I guess," I responded with little enthusiasm.

Several evenings later Tom Muller called. We met for dinner. He was twenty-one, I twenty-five, and Peter twenty-seven. The age didn't matter I told myself. I found him attractive, fun and interesting. I was fed up with Phillip Morehouse, regardless of the fact that he lived and worked in South Carolina. I never knew when I'd see or hear from him.

I invited Tom to Stone Harbor for a Saturday night. I wanted to see my parents. We enjoyed the beach, Hahn's snapper soup, and my parents. Again, I couldn't get Peter out of my mind. I kept telling myself to forget Peter and have fun, but I couldn't.

Tom invited me to Montclair, New Jersey, to meet his family the next weekend. His parents were so cordial, and we had a good time. On the way back to the City, he wanted to see my apartment. There he kissed me and wanted to make love. I hesitated and pulled back.

Ironically, Peter called at that very moment, interrupting us. "Let it ring," Tom begged.

"No...no...it might be important," I said dodging him, trying to get to the phone on the hall table. Tom heard me say the words, "Hi, Peter, can I meet you tomorrow night at around eight o'clock?" Before I could hang up the phone, Tom motioned to me that he was leaving and took off in a huff. I was glad, and even gladder that Peter wanted to see me.

*****

At eight o'clock I met Peter at his apartment; needless to say, I was nervous, but the feeling soon faded away when we sat down on the couch. That's when I opened up. I wanted to see him...to tell him what was going on...and how I felt about him. I would either blow up our relationship or I would bring us closer together. I was willing to take the chance.

"For the past two weekends I've been seeing Tom Muller, the son of friends of my parents," I said. "He just moved from Montclair to the City. Mother called, asking me if I'd like to meet him. I really didn't want to, but we went out to dinner anyway and had a good time. I was trying to forget you; thus, I invited him to Stone Harbor. That is when I realized I love you. I wished Tom had been you."

"You know it has been almost two years since we met at St. Luke's," I continued. I don't want to get hurt, Peter. I accepted his invitation to meet his parents last weekend. We had a good time but, again, Tom wasn't you. I missed you so much. On our return to the City Tom wanted to see my apartment. He wanted more than that. You couldn't have called at a better time." We both laughed. "Tom took off when he heard me say on the phone, 'Hi, Peter, can I meet you tomorrow night?'"

"Darling, I've fallen in love with you," I said. "I love you!"

Peter said he was happy that I had been frank. He was sorry he hadn't been seeing me more often, but he had been promoted to Assistant to the General Counsel at Allied. The workload was tremendous.

"YEAH...congratulations!" I bellowed out, giving him a hug.

"You know, I think I fell in love with you when you were walking down the many, many steps of Columbia University," he said. "I didn't want you to leave!"

"I wish you had told me," I said. "I, too, didn't want to go but I had classes that afternoon."

"I'm so glad you came tonight," he said and kissed me.

"Ah, that was very nice...Yes please!" I responded.

As we both had to work the next morning, Peter walked me back to my apartment at Jane Street. "I'll call you tomorrow, Sweet-Love...Goodnight," he said and kissed me again.

"I love you," I whispered in his ear.

"Yes please!" he responded and gave me a huge warm hug.

"And I better go," I said smiling. "Goodnight."

I found Peter's kisses magnetic. He always had a smile on his face...so caring and loving with such quiet demeanor. He was becoming the love of my life. I certainly was sure of that.

*****

Late that Saturday morning, Peter and I went to Midtown to Patty's Clam House at Penn Station. We adored oysters and liked the rustic atmosphere of the restaurant. As usual, the place was crowded, but we were lucky to find a picnic table with its two benches in the corner of the room away from everybody. We ordered the oysters and iced tea.

I had finished two oysters, commenting on how good they tasted, when Peter took my hand and asked, "Will you marry me?"

I almost fell off the bench, much less started to have butterflies in my stomach. "You mean you want me to become Mrs. Peter T. Hitchcock?" I asked.

Peter squeezed my hand and said, "Yes, Sweet-Love. I can't give you a ring now. It's being sized in Bronxville."

"That's OK,"I said. "Yes…yes…I'd love to become your wife." I was so excited I gave Peter the rest of my oysters as I became quite queasy, never expecting his proposal!

"I love you, Ceci. I should have told you a long time ago," said Peter.

"I love you, too, Darling. When should we get married?" I asked. "I'll need time to plan."

"How about in three months, possibly in December? That will give us three months to plan," Peter said.

"I love December. I'll have to talk to Mother. Is having the wedding in Princeton at Trinity Church ok?" I asked.

"Yes…whatever you'd like," he responded wearing a warm smile.

Peter finished my oysters, and we returned to Greenwich Village to my apartment. We were happy! Words can never describe how we felt.

*****

I called Mother. There was great excitement on the other end. I told her our plans…December at Trinity Episcopal Church and the reception at our house. Mother was fine with everything. "You'll have to come to Princeton so we can get organized. "Let me talk to Peter," she said.

"Hi, Ginny," greeted Peter happily. "We'll probably see you in Princeton next weekend."

"Congratulations…welcome to the family. I'll help as much as possible," she said and hung up the phone.

*****

Peter called his parents telling them that I had accepted his proposal…probably the wedding would take place in December in Princeton."

"Let me talk to Ceci," said his Mother. Peter handed me the phone.

"Hi, Mrs. Hitchcock. I was so surprised when he asked me," I said.

"Call me Elinor," she said. "I've known all about it for some time. Keep me up to date as to planning."

"I certainly will," I responded and handed the phone over to Peter.

"Mommy, we'll probably go to Princeton next weekend. I'll call you as soon as I know something," he said and hung up the phone.

Peter and I hugged and kissed over and over again. "To think we'll become Mr. and Mrs. Peter T. Hitchcock soon…WOW!" I said.

******

Peter went back to his apartment as he had work to do for Allied, which had moved from Rector Street to Times Square. Their new home would be in the Allied Chemical Building (now the Times Square Building). We agreed that he would come back for dinner around six o'clock.

*****

At five o'clock I began to prepare dinner: I made a spinach salad with crushed fried bacon and chopped egg; deviled the rest of the boiled eggs for hors d'oeuvres; tenderized the sirloin steak with olive oil (a trick Peter taught me) and put the washed Idaho potatoes in the oven to bake. I still had time to change clothing and make the salad dressing. We were going to celebrate!

*****

At six o'clock Peter arrived with a bouquet of the most beautiful assortment of flowers and a bottle of scotch. He knew I didn't like champagne or wine. Both were too acidic.

We sat down enjoying the deviled eggs and cocktails and talked about the wedding. We were interrupted by the phone ringing.

"Hello," I said wondering who would be calling.

"Lee, this is Phillip. Can we get together tonight?" he asked.

"Hi, Phillip," I responded, smiling at Peter. "I have good news. I'm engaged to be married."

"You are what?" he asked. "Whom are you marrying?"

"Peter Hitchcock," I answered.

"Are you sure?" he asked again.

"Absolutely!" I exclaimed emphatically.

"Congratulate Peter. He's marrying a great girl." He remarked. "Good luck." He sounded so surprised and yet sad as he hung up the phone. But this was not the end of Phillip. He called many times during our marriage! Finally, I encouraged him to try marriage.

Peter and I talked over dinner. He would ask Alan to be best man and would think about groomsmen. I decided on six attendants: Barbara, my younger sister as matron of honor; Edie; Anne, Peter's younger sister; Dana, my stepsister; my older sister, Starr; and Heather, her six-year-old daughter who was my godchild and niece, as flower girl.

First, we needed to set a date. I was to call Dr. Speers at Trinity for an appointment next Saturday; talk to Mother about having the dress rehearsal dinner Friday, as Peter's parents wanted to have a brunch at the Princeton Inn for out of towners before the wedding. We would have a busy Saturday, we agreed.

After dinner we took a walk around the neighborhood ending up at Peter's apartment. Never had we been so close and so happy in love.

*****

On September 22, 1960, Peter invited me to "The Little Place" for dinner. "SALUTE," Jimmy greeted us and led us to a table. What a memorable time we had: good food; good music; and a wonderful surprise. I received my platinum diamond engagement ring, a Hitchcock family heirloom, along with a platinum diamond guardband. Peter was quite proud of the band as he had picked it out himself! Needless to say, my ring finger on my left hand glistened and was beautiful.

*****

When the engagement announcement came out in The New York Times, I received a frightening phone call around 7:30 in the morning. I was about to go to work when the phone rang. A man's voice stated emphatically, "I'm a friend of Pete's. Please don't marry him. He's not what you think he is. I'm calling from a phone booth around the corner. I'd like to meet with you."

I hung up the phone shaking and immediately called Peter in Bronxville thinking he might be joking. Mrs. Hitchcock answered the phone. I told her the story. She put Peter right on.

"Did you just call me, Sweetheart?" I asked telling him about the phone call.

"No, Sweet-Love...some punk probably saw your engagement picture in The Times. Don't worry...just go to work," said Peter. "Besides, there isn't a phone booth around the corner from Jane Street."

"I know," I said. "That's when I became suspicious and hung up. Besides he called you Pete. I love you."

"I love you, too," he responded. "I'll call you tonight...and don't worry."

I nervously left the building and walked to NYU. Nothing like this had ever happened to me before, but I reminded myself that I was living in the City...anything could happen!

# Wedding Plans

Peter and I kept the appointment that I made with Dr. Speers at Trinity Episcopal Church the following Saturday. We learned that marriage is not allowed in an Episcopal Church during Advent or in December; however, Dr. Speers would be available the Saturday of Thanksgiving weekend, November 26, 1960. Also, we had to attend eight sessions of marriage counseling at the Church!

We called the office of the Princeton University Chapel and found that they, too, wouldn't perform a marriage in December, much less were booked in November. We, therefore, decided on November 26th after talking with our parents.

*****

Peter and I managed to make all eight sessions at Trinity. In the meantime, Mother was way ahead of me in planning, thank goodness. She presented us with a bridal book to cover the wedding. She would number the gifts, as they came in, jotting down the name and address of the gift giver. She made arrangements with a photographer to take a picture of me to announce the engagement. A picture was sent to various newspapers besides The New York Times: The Herald Tribune, The Bronxville Review Press, Princeton Town Topics, and The Chicago Daily News. My father's side of the family, the Kohlsaats, came from and lived in the Chicago area. According to Wikipedia data and dates, which were discovered by my first cousin, Kenneth Harkness, my Great-Grandfather, Christian Cecil Kohlsaat, was appointed by President William McKinley in 1899 to the United States Court of Appeals for the Seventh Circuit of the Northern District of Illinois.

*****

One Saturday I met Mother at Penn Station in Manhattan. We had such fun picking out bridesmaid dresses in the Garment District. I wanted an all-white wedding; thus, we decided on a short white velveteen dress with a v-neckline suitable for all five girls. The same dress would be made for Heather, my niece. The company was willing to make white velveteen muffs for each bridesmaid along with white velveteen headbands decorated with ostrich feathers. We had such success!

*****

I was to be the eleventh member to wear the family heirloom bridal gown. It was creamy satin with an overblouse and apron of Alencon lace. The heirloom cap held my veil of Rose Point lace with a long trailing train. I had only three fittings to adjust the apron and length of the dress, thank goodness.

*****

Peter decided on his groomsmen: Alan was to be best man. Ushers would be Gaylord Hitchcock, Peter's brother; Keith McLean; Ned Boody; George Childs; Dick Bauer and Mike Morgan, my stepbrother. He asked Bill Knox but he had already accepted the invitation to be in another wedding. We were disappointed. Bill begged us to change the date but we decided to stay with the 26th.

Peter also met with his groomsmen in the City to pick out the wedding cutaways. They were elegant and quite aristocratic! The waistcoats with peeked lapels were dark Oxford gray, the trousers black with silvertone stripes, and the ascots and gloves pearl gray.

*****

After meeting with Dr. Speers at Trinity one Saturday, we walked to "Renwicks" on Nassau Street, the main street in Princeton, for lunch. We then went on to "The Cummins Shop" to pick out our china pattern and various gift ideas for The Bridal Registry. The store would send a list to Mother and Peter's parents. We had such fun!

*****

Much to our surprise Town and Country magazine contacted us asking for three of our best wedding photographs for their "Wedding Day" section. The picture would come out in the February, 1961 issue of the magazine. They would send us copies.

*****

Our last chore for Mother and me was to pick out flowers from a local florist. The bridesmaids' muffs and ostrich headbands had arrived several days earlier. We asked the florist to add to the muffs white gardenias intertwined with ivy; white rose petals for my flower girl, along with lily-of-the-valley on her headband; white carnations for our fathers; white rose boutonnieres for the groom, best man, and groomsmen.

My bouquet would have several gardenias, white orchids, and stephanotis; lastly, for our two mothers and grandmothers orchid corsages.

*****

It was hard to believe but four hundred and twenty-three people accepted the wedding invitations – and I wanted a small wedding! Trinity Church could seat all of the guests but Mike, my stepfather, was wondering about 36 Mercer Street. Could it hold so many people? He, therefore, asked the Fire Chief of Princeton for his opinion. The consensus was only two hundred could attend the reception because of the age of the house. People from out of town, family and very close friends would be invited. The rest could only attend the church ceremony.

*****

We had a wonderful surprise; Mother's sister, Aunt Margaret McLean, took care of our Kirk sterling silver pattern. The eight-piece place settings with my initials, "CHK" were given by family members!

******

As our wedding approached, I took the week off to help Mother as Thanksgiving was that Thursday. What a special and fun time we shared preparing for the festive weekend! During this time, I also wrote "thank you" notes for gifts we had received; noting to each that we were looking forward to seeing them at the wedding or we were sorry they couldn't make it.

At the receiving line during the reception, we overheard, "It's the first time we've ever received a 'thank you' note before the wedding!" I felt very proud, as did Peter, but happy to get the notes out of the way, as I had to work after the honeymoon. Needless to say, I went through boxes of note paper!

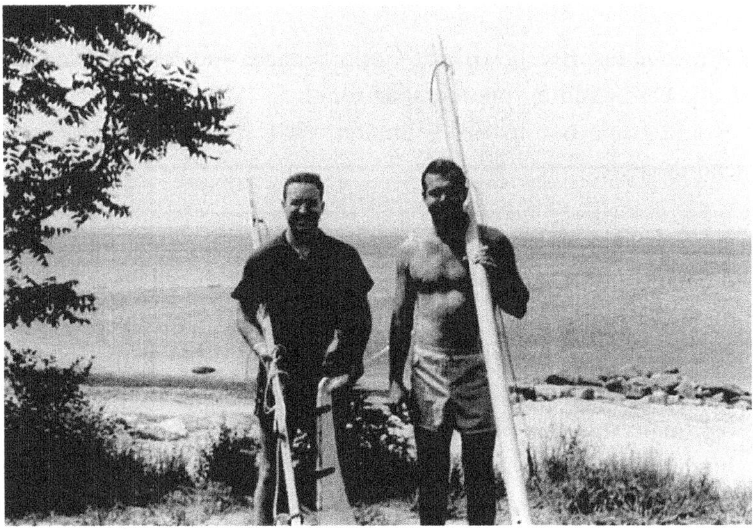

Peter and Alan in Bayville L.I. 1960

# The Duck and I

We had picture-perfect weather for the wedding – a cloudless blue sky, warm sunlight, and a slight breeze. Peter, Alan, and Edie arrived early Friday afternoon, as did two ushers, Keith McLean and Dick Bauer. We decided to walk up to "Renwicks" on Nassau Street for a quick hamburger. What a fun and hilarious time we had – old friends getting together!

Peter, I, and most of the bridal party gathered at Trinity Church at five pm for the rehearsal. Gaylord and Anne would arrive with Horace and Elinor Hitchcock early tomorrow morning before the brunch, along with two ushers. Thankfully, Mother had made arrangements with friends to put up the whole wedding party.

It felt wonderful, almost magical, to be walking up the aisle with Mike following the five attendants, and knowing that Peter was waiting for me at the altar. The attendants were to form a line to the left of the altar, the groomsmen to the right. I said to Mike, "Can you believe this!" "Oh, yes," he said. "You're marrying a fine boy. We like him. He'll take good care of you." I knew he was right.

As we approached the altar, Barbara, my matron of honor, was to straighten my train, if needed, and to take my bouquet. Mike was to join Mother in the front pew along with other relatives. I caught Peter smiling. He was as happy as I was. He looked so adorably handsome standing next to Alan, his best man. This time tomorrow we will be husband and wife!

Peter walked over and stood by my side. "I love you," he whispered taking my hand. "I love you, too," I whispered back, squeezing his hand. After Dr. Speers talked about vows, Peter and I marched down the aisle followed by the bridal party. The ushers then returned to escort Mother, my two grandmothers, and other relatives.

We thanked Dr. Speers who told us that he would not be able to join us at the reception tomorrow. We then headed across the street to the house. Mother did a good job finding accommodations for the bridal party. Everyone got settled in nearby homes. I drove Edie to the Whitman's where she changed clothes. We returned to 36 Mercer Street. By then, Peter and Alan were at the house. I ran upstairs and changed into a beautiful winter white wool, sleeveless dress dotted with rhinestones and my new white satin heels. Grandmother Myers, much to my surprise, gave me as wedding presents: the dress; a gorgeous going away, green-purple wool suit; a lovely purple coat with a fox collar; and an eighteen karat gold bracelet she had bought in Switzerland.

At seven pm we all gathered for a fun dinner with wonderful friends. Laughter filled the room as we enjoyed cocktails and hors d'oeuvres. Mother had hired extra help which enabled Mike and her to join in the fun. We chuckled over jokes, storytelling, and reminiscing over school days.

A delicious buffet was served, consisting of sliced baked ham and turkey tetrazzini, tossed salad, and a variety of hard and soft rolls. For dessert there was as an assortment of cheesecake.

After dinner I asked Alan, "Where is Edie?"

"She went upstairs to see your wedding presents," he responded.

"Sweet-Love, you'll be shocked, but happy, over the things we were given," I said to Peter. "Would you all like to join us?"

"Cecil, I can't get over all that you've received," shouted Edie from the second floor. "Your mother did a fantastic job of arranging everything."

"Did you hear Edie, Mother?" I asked. "Thank you so much. I don't know what we would have done without you!" I kissed her on the cheek.

We all joined Edie upstairs in the flowered wallpapered bedroom with the large fireplace. There were eleven tables adorned with white tablecloths. Mother had put pieces of silver on one table, crystal and cut glass on another, stainless steel serving pieces along with entertainment equipment, lovely china lamps with silk shades, plenty of bowls, and so forth – in all 423 presents!

We decided it was time to turn in. I kissed Peter goodnight." This time tomorrow night, Darling!" I said. "I can't wait Sweet-Love," said Peter. "I love you." "I love you, too," I said. "Goodnight!"

Just as I was climbing the steps to go to bed, Keith McLean came out of the back bedroom. "Would you like a sip of brandy?" he asked. "Oh, no thanks…I'm getting married tomorrow!" I responded happily.

*****

The Hitchcock's brunch at eleven thirty am at the Princeton Inn, right around the corner from Mercer Street, turned out to be an enormous success. Peter and I held hands as we entered the ballroom. We could hear, "Here they come!" It was very exciting, even though we knew it was bad luck to see each other on the big day. We also were proud to have the brunch at the Inn. According to www.princeton.edu, there is a fascinating history of the Princeton Inn. It was "built in 1924-25. Was a gracious rambling hotel. On the rear terrace, overlooking the pond of Springdale Golf Course, where the British had made a temporary stand during the Battle of Princeton, guests could sip a cocktail and listen to music of the carillon float down from the Cleveland Tower. Now the college occupies the main building at the Inn, as well as the former employees' quarters called the Annex, and a new building opened in 1971, the addition. Four hundred and forty undergraduates live in these facilities. On the terrace where waiters in formal dress once served mint juleps." The Inn is now called Forbes College.

The self-serve buffet was inviting with its decorations of boiled red lobsters resting on ice chips, surrounded by dishes of food, fresh trimmed artichokes with bunches of kale and parsley. I couldn't eat, as I had no appetite. Instead, I decided to say "hello" to our guests. How happy I was to see Peter's parents talking to Grandmother Myers, my mother's mother. Grandfather had died four years earlier of Parkinson's Disease. I thanked Elinor and Horace Hitchcock for the lovely brunch. Peter joined me. Soon after, we left the Inn to get ready for the two-thirty wedding.

I made sure that I followed the "good luck" wedding tradition: something new – my white satin white shoes; something old – my dress; something borrowed – a dime from Mike; something blue – a piece of blue ribbon from one of my gifts. The ribbon and dime went into my shoe.

I told Mother I felt funny walking across the street to Trinity Church from 36 Mercer Street in a bridal dress. Suppose I tore the train? Could I go around the block in a limousine? Mother agreed but insisted that the bridesmaids walk across the street!

*****

The shiny black, stretch limousine arrived around two-ten and took me around the block. The family never let me forget this in the future!

Just before the ceremony outside the church, I asked my bridesmaids if I looked all right? There wasn't a peep from anyone. They all were engrossed in each other and their own selves. Mike, who would walk me up the aisle, thought I looked lovely, which reassured me.

Mendelssohn's Wedding March from "A Midsummer Night's Dream" began to play. For some reason I wasn't nervous. I knew I'd see Peter at the altar. It was a long walk up the aisle, but I was happy we would be united. In a way, it was hard to believe I was in church in a wedding dress, surrounded by so many people, and getting married. We didn't forget a word repeating our vows; however, I was somewhat troubled with the words, "until death do us part." I don't know what I'd do if I lost Peter!

*****

Little did I know, until I heard it at the reception, that my Uncle Frank, my father's sister's husband, was listening to the Army-Navy game throughout the ceremony! I didn't care really, as Peter slipped away several times during the reception to find out the game's score. I believe Navy won!

*****

The receiving line took at least two hours to greet two hundred guests. Peter and I then celebrated with sipping sparkling champagne from the bridal cup between toasts and cutting the cake. We tried not to make a mess feeding each other a bite from the three-tiered cake! I remember Alan's toast: "Peter and I met Ceci while at Columbia Law School and she at St. Luke's School of Nursing, through my wife, Edie, who was also a student. Ceci had just lost her beloved dog, "Pooh Bear," a great loss to her. By meeting Peter, her life changed. They fell in love almost immediately...here's to a great couple. Edie and I wish you a wonderful future together with years of happiness and far beyond."

Soon after, and halfway up our stairway, I threw my bouquet. Dana Morgan, my step-sister, caught it. She and Fred were married a year later!

Alan and Edie would drive us to Idlewild International Airport (now The John F. Kennedy International Airport), before taking the flight to Nassau. We had wanted to go to Bermuda but were told it wasn't a good time of year to visit because of the weather.

We stayed at The Sheraton Hotel at the airport for the night as our flight to Nassau was the next morning. The room was very comfortable overlooking the airport's runway. We were tired from all the excitement, but absolutely overjoyed to be married. It didn't take long for us to be in each other's arms and fall into the world of Inanity, as Mr. and Mrs. Peter T. Hitchcock. Words are so inadequate to express how we felt.

Later, we took the elevator down to the dining room. I was so hungry as I hadn't eaten all day; however, I made a foolish mistake! I ordered duck, a favorite of mine. I should have had what Peter had – roast beef. Never have I been so sick all night. Keith McLean, one of Peter's ushers, had given Peter a pint of brandy before leaving the house. Thinking a sip might settle my stomach, Peter suggested I try a taste. That, too, was a mistake. I spent most of the night in and out of the bathroom.

Alan sent a card on our twentieth anniversary:

"You are to be heartily congratulated having set what must be the Easterly Regional record for longevity of having been married to the same person, and (from one who knows whereof he speaks) for sticking together through thick and thin and most recently (I fear) thin.

ADVICE:
Avoid having duck for dinner on your anniversary eve.
That I remembered all on my own.
Alan"

As it was Sunday, we couldn't fine an aspirin any place…not in the Sheraton, the airport, the plane, or the Royal Victoria Hotel in Nassau. However, I made it through the day drinking Coca-Cola and eating lightly!

We called our parents before leaving on the morning ten-thirty PanAm flight to thank them again for a beautiful wedding. They were extremely pleased that we called.

*****

Our honeymoon was wonderful. We had fun exploring Nassau, the Island of New Providence: its Fort Fincastle; the Old Prison; the Princess Margaret Hospital; a trip on "The Tropic Bird" to Athol Island, Bahamas; a trip in a glass-bottom boat to Paradise Beach on Hog Island (now Paradise Island); we visited Bay Street with its shops and open-air markets; the Straw Market Place, where I bargained for a handmade brown and beige purse and hat to match. Peter said I was the best bargainer he had ever seen!

The Royal Victoria was a beautiful tropical hotel. Unfortunately, we had a noisy visitor in our room for several nights. Peter finally tossed shoes at the closet – enough was enough! Out came a mouse in the moonlit room and disappeared.

Then, late one afternoon, I decided to collect shells along the water's edge for Edie's lamp. We returned to our hotel room to change clothes for dinner. I put the shells on the bedside table. We then left, taking the elevator to the first floor to the dining room, where we enjoyed the buffet and music by the Royal Victorians. Peter and I loved to dance. It was fun trying to swing to Calypso rhythms.

After dinner, upon paying the bill, I caught the waiter looking down into Peter's wallet. I gently kicked Peter under the table to let him know what the waiter was doing. He looked at me and then up at the surprised waiter. We gave no tip that night!

Returning to the room, we found the shells very much alive! They traveled around the bedside table, up the glass-based lamp, and down on the wideboard floor. We laughed until tears fell from our eyes. "What should we do?" I asked Peter. "I have an idea." It was too late to return them to their natural habitat. We would have to wait until morning; thus, I placed them in the bathtub and covered it with towels for the night. The next morning we returned them to the beach after a delightful breakfast, which was in the hotel's Garden Patio.

We left for the States soon after. It had been a restful and fun honeymoon. Gradually we moved my things into Peter's apartment in the evenings, as we both worked. My landlady refused to return my security deposit at Jane Street. Peter tried using his lawyer's charm to no avail. We were annoyed as $110.00 in 1960 was a lot of money! The day after Christmas, using the Vauxhall, we picked up the wedding presents in Princeton. At last, we could call 133 W. 12th Street home.

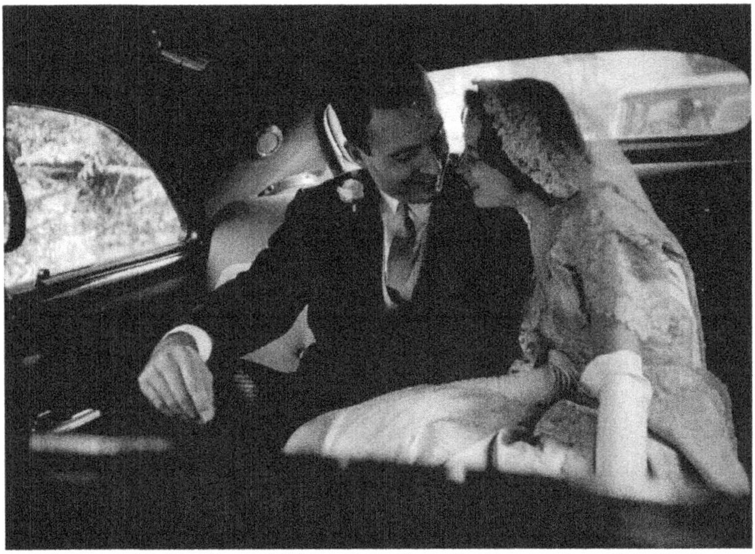

Mr. and Mrs. Peter Tilden Hitchcock, November 26, 1960

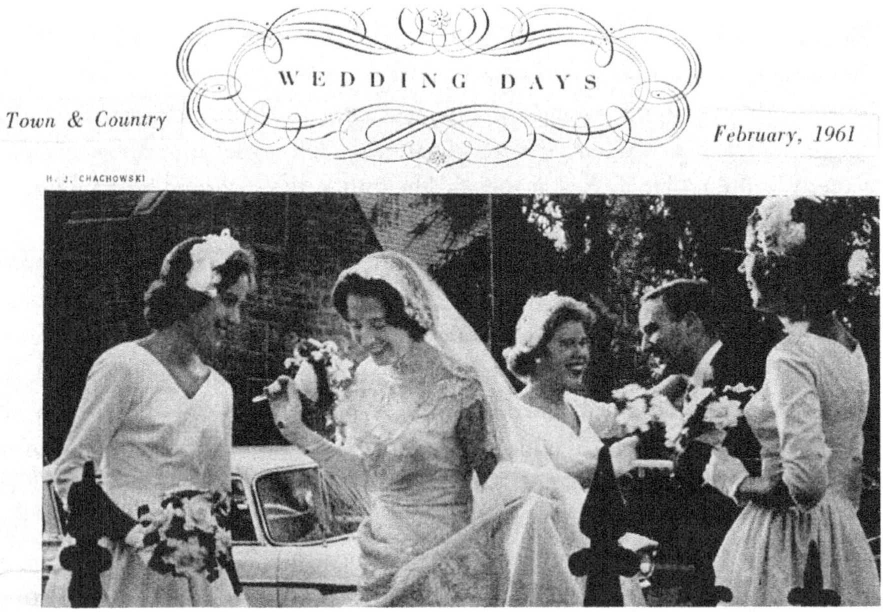


"Wedding Days" in TOWN & COUNTRY, February 1961

# Part Three: Married Life

## Keeping in Touch

Married life proved to be amazingly happy, as it is said the first year of marriage is the hardest year to get along with your spouse! It was a thrill to become a couple for we had never lived with each other. We had a few spats trying to get used to each other's ways. But never once did we wake up grumpy or unwilling to talk. We always ended up in each other's arms entering the world of Inanity.

If you can get through the first year, I believe, you're on the right path to a healthy marriage. As it turned out, 1961 was a busy year for us in spite of the fact that Peter had begun to travel.

How wonderful the Hitchcocks were to accept me into the family. Gaylord, now a junior in high school, I got to know well. Anne, Peter's sister, followed in her mother's footsteps by going to Vassar College (Elinor had graduated in 1924). Anne and I became good friends. She also loved New Boston.

There were birthdays and holiday get-togethers at Avon Road, and meetings and partying with Peter's friends, namely, "The Seedy Six:" six boys who grew up together. As for Christmas and Thanksgiving, Peter and I rotated each with our parents, which seemed to work out well.

We were invited by Edie and Alan to Bayville, Long Island, several times, where they rented a carriage house right on the water's edge, a part of a magnificent estate set back from the Sound. The boys loved to clam, boat, and fish, while Edie and I had fun cooking their catch besides enjoying each other's company.

We also had a good time with Ned Boody (one of our ushers) and his wife, Mary. They invited us to their home in Little Silver, New Jersey, and took us to Quogue, Long Island, where we relaxed on the beach. Peter tried to water ski with little success. It is a great sport that looks easy but isn't. As Peter said, "At least I tried!"

We did fit in trips to New Boston. As promised, Peter took me up to Ned's log cabin on Snow Mountain from Mrs. Perkins' house. What a hike! How Ned got the piano up there had to have been a major project. The view from the bungalow was outstanding showing the stand of trees, where the two tennis courts once stood, surrounded by 250 acres, divided by stone walls, with mountains in the background. We couldn't see our house as it was hidden by a line of trees.

We met Mrs. Perkins one afternoon for a short visit as she was ill in bed. She died soon after – what a lovely lady: kind, graceful, and happy to meet me finally. Elinor Hitchcock must have kept in touch with her as she knew all about us. I hated to leave New Boston each time we went up there: so peaceful, serene, and private.

*****

On August 10, 1961, Peter's father, Horace Hitchcock, died of a massive heart attack while entering the building for work in the City. Charles R. Cox, my boss, knew Horace well; thus, I was given a week off from work. We stayed in Bronxville to be with Elinor. After the funeral, we both commuted to the City to our jobs for a while. NYU's "75 Million Campaign" came to a close. I transferred to the University's Student Credit and Loan Department in charge of loans and scholarships. I enjoyed working with the students, thank goodness. Soon Peter would spend more time traveling than at home.

*****

Peter was promoted to Special Corporate Counsel responsible for all legal matters of the International Division for Allied, including negotiations, organization and operation of foreign joint venture projects. He worked with subsidiaries in Europe, Latin America and the Far East—had performed a similar function for the Fiber Division. Life certainly became chaotic for us!

In October, 1961, Peter was sent to Frankfurt, Germany, then on to New Delhi, India, to work on a nitrogen proposed urea joint venture. That kept him there for four weeks.

The whole time we wrote each other every night. I was thankful that my job kept me busy. I also had extra time fixing up our apartment in the evenings if I didn't have to work. Frequently, I went to visit Peter's mother in Bronxville and my parents in Princeton on weekends. Peter and I missed each other terribly but our letters kept us going. They exemplified our love for each other and showed how wonderful and bright Peter was. His letters were warm, loving and quite literary. I will quote a few here:

> October 1961
> "Hotel Frankfurter Hof
> Frankfurt Am Main
> Frankfurt, Germany

My little Sweetie-spoose-darling:

Your cable arrived this afternoon bringing you that much closer for a moment. Speaking of feeling close, my tummy reaches out to you every time I read your letter, which warmed me with love while I was on the plane, and gave me a nice Ceci-filled sleep. I hope my cable reached you without delay.

We have finished our business here, and are getting ready to leave first thing tomorrow for New Delhi. Even after only two days I feel sad about leaving Frankfurt and the pleasant countryside surrounding it. A number of times I thought how much I want to be able to show you these places sometime.

Every time I walk down these streets I wish you could be alongside, (needless to say, these are not the only times I have wished you were here with me). I'll write again Sunday, meanwhile please take care of My Darling.

I love you,

Peter"

October 8th

"ASHOKA HOTELSunday,

NEW DEHLI

My Darling:

We arrived here about six in the morning, and napped for about five hours, after which we had lunch and then drove around New Delhi. Our sightseeing included a mosque, and a cremation place, where Hindu corpses are burned. A rather grim, bad-smelling place, but fortunately no action was going on at the time.

The view from my window is fascinating, with large-domed buildings looming up in the background, occasional flights of ravens in the sky giving a weird, almost other-worldly touch to the scene. I have gotten several pictures of this view already.

I deeply wish you could be here now not only to share these strange sights with me, but far more because of the comfort and happiness your presence would bring. Being away from you makes me realize this even more.

The cable went off this afternoon to Princeton and will catch you there, I hope. If not, your mother can let you know it arrived. I'll write again tomorrow.

I love you, Sweetie,

Peter"

October 11, 1961

"ASHOKA HOTEL

NEW DELHI

My Darling:

I received yesterday your letters of October 4th and 5th, both of which pulled my tummy thousands of miles, right to 133 W. 12th St. I am so very glad you are doing well, and hope the weekend festivities at Princeton were fun.

We talked with the Indians yesterday, also with the American Commercial attaché at the Embassy. This morning I am to talk with the lawyer for Andhra Sugars (the Indian company) and have been up since 6 am getting ready. We are scheduled to go to Hyderabad tonight for about a week, after which I expect to go to Bombay to talk with the lawyers, then back to New Delhi.

I hate having this letter sound matter of fact, but you know I don't feel that way. Last night I dropped off to sleep imagining that you were snuggled up next to me. Don't I wish that were so.

I love My Darling,

Peter"

October 21, 1961

"TAJ MAHAL HOTEL

BOMBAY, INDIA

My Darling,

Thank you for your cable, which I have just received. With all this back-country moving about, it's the only way I can be sure that you're all right.

Bombay is a large, cosmopolitan city, with a climate which is currently pretty much like New York in August. It's humid climate-wise, dry otherwise, although I have secured my foreigner's liquor permit, a most impressive document.

I miss you very much, and have been dreaming of you. Last night we went to a Princeton football game – I never could figure out who Princeton's opponent was, but I think we won. Anyway, you and I had a good time together.

The rest of our group is in Hyderabad, but I am being entertained and looked-after by some people here, and I find it most relaxing. I expect to go back to New Delhi by the middle of next week.

I love you and miss you,

Peter"

Peter found out that he had to start scotch taping his letters closed with an inked "X" for privacy. He asked me to do the same. Below I have quoted a few of his loving and interesting letters:

November 1, 1961

"ASHOKA HOTEL

NEW DELHI

My Darling:

I received your nine letters on Friday (the hotel had some difficulty locating them), and felt as though I had actually been with you over the past two weeks. In my mind, you had been with me during that time, but your letters seemed to enable me to share in your life.

We have been quite busy during the days, with conferences and preparation of studies and reports. The only times we have gotten out of the Ashoka have been to go to the offices of Indian Government officials. We are going to see the Taj Mahal before we go, however.

November 2$^{nd}$

Everything is pretty well cleaned up, now. We even got to go to the Taj Mahal yesterday. Dale Gooden and I have been able to book ourselves on a BOAC flight leaving Delhi at10 p.m. tomorrow (Friday) and arriving in London Saturday. Will get some sleep there, and try to get a flight to New York the next day.

I miss you Sweetie and am terribly happy to be almost by your side (timewise, anyway).

I love my little Sweetie-poose,

Peter"

Upon Peter's return from India, we gave an open house at our new home, 133 W. 12th Street, inviting friends from the City and Bronxville. Peter called from the office, just as guests arrived, to say that he had to work. He would join us around ten pm! Disappointed, I asked our good friend, Bill Knox, to bartend while I entertained our guests as best I could. I was so thankful that I had made a large assortment of hors d'oeuvres earlier that day as it would be a late evening. All went well, but I was happy to see Peter at ten pm.

I kept telling myself I had better get used to this kind of life...Peter working late at night and traveling so much. We absolutely adored each other and hated to be apart. I was proud of him though and wanted him to be successful in his career whatever it would take.

He was traveling within the United States at the moment...no trip to India as yet! We kept our fingers crossed. Each time he announced he had to leave, I would pack his suitcase and slip a note inside his briefcase:

> "My Darling:
>
> I hope Allied Chemical appreciates you as much as I do. You are such a hardworking, brilliant lawyer. I am so proud of you.
>
> Have a good trip, and may God bring you safely back to me. Remember I am in your pocket.
>
> I love you,
>
> Your Spoose"

When we could, Peter and I always managed to fit in short weekend trips to New Boston, visit our families, or tailgate with friends at a Princeton football game. We did attend Exeter's 81st Annual Dinner at the Biltmore where we sat at table 22 with the 1949 class. Peter and his classmates had fun reminiscing over the good old days.

We were quite surprised that Keith McLean, an usher and Princeton classmate, married Mary Vaughn (the girl at Edie and Alan's wedding who said she and Peter were almost engaged!). We received an invitation to dinner at their apartment one Saturday night. Upon arriving we were asked to put our coats on the bed in the master bedroom. There were mirrors all over the place. Peter kidded Keith who confessed that Mary liked mirrors when making love! We had such a lovely time with the other five couples who had been invited also. In the future the McLeans had two children. Keith called Peter one night saying that Mary had confessed the children weren't his. He immediately took off for California and committed suicide. We were heartbroken as we had lost a dear friend.

I remember well in the early 60's there was an English rock band, called the Beatles, founded by John Lennon. The band consisted of Paul McCartney, George Harrison, Ringo Starr, and John. Their music became influential and so popular that the Beatles were invited to the United States and introduced to America on the Ed Sullivan Show.

*****

On January 22, 1963, Peter returned to India for a four-week stay. I quote a love letter he sent to me mentioning that negotiations were going slowly:

> February 3, 1963
> "ASHOKA HOTEL
> NEW DELHI
>
> My Sweet-Darling:
>
> Your letters of the 29th and 30th arrived today, bringing a little (too little) bit of you right into my room.
>
> Yesterday Dale and I took several hours off to take a drive to Faridabad, a town some twenty miles south of New Delhi, in Punjab state. The only thing to look at was a reservoir lake, but we had a very pleasant lunch at a hotel (really a newly built motel) called the 'Holiday Inn,' a familiar name. It appears to me that its room clientele must at least partially be made up of dirty-weekenders. At least it's an ideal spot for that. Wish you were here so that we could pretend.
>
> The time schedule is still up in the air, dependent mainly on how talks with the government proceed. Certainly I do not have

the remotest hope of getting out of here before the end of February, but certainly will do my best.

Do take care of my little Cutie-Sweetie,

I love you,

Peter"

We continued to write love letters every night to keep us close and help the time pass quickly. Peter hoped that I might join him in Europe, but he had to wait for more progress in negotiations with the Indians; however, two weeks later I received a Western Union telegram stating that he and Dale were on their way home. They had stopovers, where Peter sent postcards from Bangkok, Thailand; Manila, Philippines; and Honolulu, Hawaii, which they loved. Needless to say, when they arrived in New York City, I was overjoyed to see my darling husband at last, as was Judy with Dale.

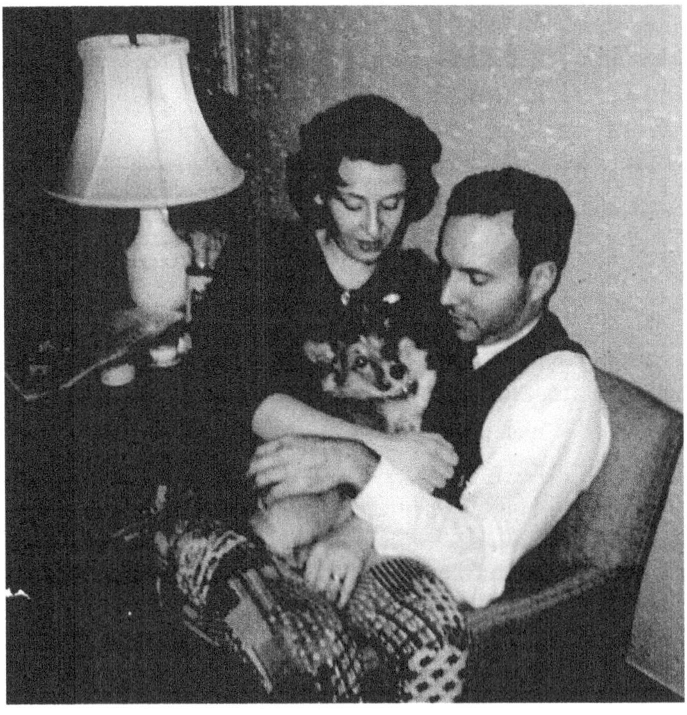

# The Trip to Bermuda

My 32nd birthday was one that I will never forget! Peter came home from work that night with a vase full of colorful, spring flowers and announced that he had made reservations at "The Little Place." We do something special on birthdays to celebrate.

"You always remember, Sweetheart. The flowers are beautiful…thank you…you're so good to me," I said giving him a kiss. "Yes…I'd love to go to "The Little Place."

"Good…we have a few more surprises ahead of us, Sweet-Darling," he said kissing me back.

Upon our arrival, Jimmy welcomed us at the restaurant's door. "SALUTE," he said shaking our hands. "How have you been?"

"Doing well…thanks," Peter responded pulling him aside. I wondered what all the whispering was about. While Jimmy disappeared into the kitchen, we found a table for two and sat down. Peter took my hand and said, "Sweet-Love, I love you so much!"

"What are you up to?" I queried with a warm grin.

"Well, since we can't meet in Europe this year, I thought the next best thing would be to take a trip to Paget, Bermuda. I talked to Bill Knox, who called The Coral Beach and Tennis Club, since he and Betty are members, and in return I received this," he said taking a note out of the pocket of his suit coat and handing it to me.

"The Board of Governors of The Coral Beach and Tennis Club is pleased to extend the privileges of the Club to Mr. and Mrs. Peter Hitchcock for the period of May 25-June2nd, 1963."

Sweetheart, I'm flabbergasted…how absolutely, positively fantastic. It is beyond anything I could imagine but then you're always full of surprises!" I said squeezing his hand. "Darling, I'm the luckiest person in the world to be married to such an amazing man…precious, caring, and sagacious! I love you so much."

"And I love you, too, Sweet-Love," he said smiling, his eyes sparkling. A waiter served our favorites for dinner: Seafood Fra Diavolo over linguine for Peter and Eggplant Parmesan for me. Jimmy began to serenade us with his operatic arias. It was quite a birthday celebration!

But it wasn't over yet! After we finished dinner, a waiter returned with a small, fancily decorated cake, accompanied by two other waiters and Jimmy. While they and other guests in the restaurant sang "Happy Birthday," Peter and

I quickly put our rings on the candle and made a wish…I then blew! "Thank you, Jimmy," I said and turned to Peter. "I bet we wished the same thing!"

We headed back to 12th Street excited, talking about Bermuda. "I should be able to take the time off from work," I commented. "I have vacation days, and it isn't a busy time of year for our office. Let's keep our fingers crossed!"

Arriving back at the apartment, Peter gave me a big hug and a magnetic kiss that lasted quite a while. "We're being enticed by Lethe, Bacchus, and Morpheus – Gods of oblivion, wine, and dreams. Let us drift happily into Inanity," Peter whispered and led me into the bedroom.

"Yes please," I agreed. There was a spark of intense chemistry between the two of us. We absolutely adored being in each other's arms. Peter was a great lover…always putting me first…gentle and caring. I knew he loved me which made me feel so secure and happy.

*****

The next day, Dorothy McDonald at the office was thrilled for us about the trip. "There wouldn't be a problem taking the time off," she said. I immediately called Peter at his office. "We're going to Bermuda!" I said excitedly. Our wishes had come true!

*****

In the early afternoon, on May 25th, we arrived by PanAm in Bermuda, having had lunch on the plane. We took a taxi to The Coral Beach and Tennis Club which was on twenty-one lush acres and overlooked the South Shore of Paget Parish. The calm blue-green, rolling sea brushed the beautiful pristine pink, sandy beach. The Club, itself, was lovely in every way but formal – members only. It encompassed cottages, suites, and rooms in wings of the Clubhouse. Welcomed by the Concierge, we were led to our corner suite #2 which consisted of a bedroom, bath, and terrace. Breakfast would be delivered to our room, if ordered the night before, a box lunch also.

After unpacking our clothes we changed into our bathing suits and made our way to the outside terraces…one was the Beach Terrace, the swimmer's bar, which served informal lunch and dinner. We were told that the Main Club, Patio, and Dining Terrace were not to be used when in bathing attire – jackets, ties, and long trousers were to be worn during the dinner hour! Every Tuesday there was a barbecue with Red Smith and his calypso music and on other evenings formal dancing to Freddie Chapman and his " B'MUDIANS."

Peter and I walked down the many steps to the beach. We took a long walk, holding hands, as we waded through the warm water to relax after the flight. Upon returning to the Club we dressed for dinner. I was thankful I had brought several long dresses and cocktail outfits. The headwaiter led us to our table assigned to us for the week. Our waiter was very sophisticated but amicable...the menu lavish, our meal gourmet and delicious. We did sign up for breakfast to be delivered the next morning.

At nine am sharp there was a rap on the door, announcing our food had arrived. I hurriedly put on my robe, Peter his trousers, and greeted the boy. The waiter, a young college graduate, said, "Good Morning," as he walked out to the terrace, putting the tray on the table. Peter thanked him, and we went out to the porch with our night clothes on. The terrace was that private. The scrambled eggs, bacon, fresh fruit, toast, and coffee were most enjoyable. It was certainly a wonderful way to start the day. Being waited upon made us feel like a king and queen, a grand experience; however, we soon found out that we had company...sparrows! As we ate, the birds sat on the terrace wall eventually flying over to our table waiting for a bite to eat! One even landed on Peter's coffee cup and tried to indulge. It was hysterical!

After breakfast we took a walk on the beach, which we started to do every morning during our stay, and then rented motor bikes...always being reminded to drive on the left side of the road (Island guests were not allowed to rent cars).

Peter and I had an amazing time – not a minute was wasted. We motor biked to Flatts Inlet. There we visited the Government Aquarium, Museum, and Tropical Bird Sanctuary...had lunch at the Coral Island Club on Harrington Sound. Later, we tooted across the Causeway of St. George, visiting Fort St. Catherine, which was fascinating, especially to Peter, a history buff. We saw the crown jewels in replica and historical dioramas. St. George, we learned, was the original capital of the Colony and the site of the first English settlers in the Islands.

Another day we went to the Penthouse Club in Hamilton for lunch after doing a great deal of shopping earlier. We purchased duty free gifts for family members and ourselves. At The English Shop, Peter insisted that I buy a tiger, two-piece bathing suit, a reminder of Princeton. We then went on to H.A. & E. Smith, LTD. where we looked at Egg Codallers which Peter used in England when he was in the Navy. "A Codaller is a ceramic container with a string attached to the top – add melted butter inside, along with an egg or two, and seasonings. With top on tight, drop the Codaller in boiling water – Abracadabra!"Peter laughed putting his arm around my waist- "You have poached eggs. You'll love them, Sweet-Love."

"How ingenious!" I said. "Let's buy four...two for us and two for your mother."

"Good idea," Peter agreed.

Taking advantage of Trimingham's sales, we bought scarves, paisley and silk ties, and a pair of coral-colored Bermuda shorts for Peter. Splurging, he selected a London Fog zipper-lined raincoat at A.S. Cooper, and at Cecile Maison Francaise four bottles of his favorite aftershave, Royal Lime Lotion. Much to our surprise, we were also able to buy a place setting of our Lenox Kingsley bone china pattern for much less than in Trenton, New Jersey, where it was made! Liquor was half price; thus, we bought several bottles of liqueur and a case of Chivas Regal, ending up paying Customs for extra weight!

Early one morning, after a quick walk on the beach, we took our bikes on the ferry, the CORONA, to Somerset crossing The Great Sound to Watford Bridge and on to Ely's Harbour. There the water is shallow for small boats and picnickers. It is said that the Somerset Bridge is the smallest drawbridge in the World! Ending our adventure, we had lunch at the 21 Club in Hamilton. That day was great fun.

We continued our journey of exploration late one afternoon. We motor biked out to Gibb's Hill Lighthouse in Southampton. There we climbed eight flights or 185 steps (322 feet) to the top. The view was extraordinary of the Little and Great Sound, Southampton, Somerset, Paget, and Hamilton. We learned that the lighthouse began flashing its beam to seafaring men on May 1, 1846. It was built of cast iron, as steel was not available at that time.

The day before we were to leave for New York, we took a long walk on the beach investigating the Elbow Beach Surf Club, a beautiful and very popular hotel. We then tooted to Hamilton to the highly recommended smorgasbord luncheon at the Ace of Clubs. I'm glad we went, as the food was plentiful and delicious. We then continued to motor bike a little more on the winding Island roads, before handing in the bikes at the Coral Beach.

Returning to our suite to change, we decided to have dinner outside on the starlit Dining Terrace. We danced the night away to the music of Freddie Chapman and his "B'MUDIANS." Dancing was a wonderful way of keeping close. As a result, we found our love growing stronger and stronger!

The next morning, before we boarded our PanAm flight, Peter bought a copy of Bermuda's The Royal Gazette Weekly newspaper which he wanted to read on the plane. Sadly, the headlines announced that eighty-one year old Pope John XXIII had stomach cancer and was being given last rites. St. Peter's Square, in Rome, Italy, was crowded by the faithful waiting for news.

We will miss Bermuda! There was much more to see, and different cuisines to try – but we will be back, we agreed.

Returning to the States, we knew another trip to India was inevitable, but we kept our fingers crossed that it wouldn't be too soon; nevertheless, at Allied Chemical Peter began to work overtime trying to resolve issues with the Indians.

*****

It was on November 22, 1963 that I had a late morning appointment at the beauty parlor. I remember calling Peter at the office.

"Hi, Darling," I said. "I'm having my hair cut. I'll be leaving the office shortly."

"Don't have it cut too short," he said. "I like you in long hair…my sexy, beautiful Wife!"

"I'm just having my hair styled," I laughed, reassuring him. As the beauty parlor wasn't busy, I was taken immediately. I looked forward to the massaging shampoo, a favorite part of going to the hairdresser, but no sooner had I sat down when the classical music in the background was silenced.

> *We interrupt this program to inform you that at 12 noon John F. Kennedy was assassinated as he, John Connelly, and Jackie Kennedy rode in the motorcade in Dallas, Texas. Connelly was hurt but Jackie seems to be all right.*

I felt like crying. "We have just lost the greatest 35th President," I remarked to Laura, the beautician. "Yes," she said. "He did so much for our country. Who would do such a thing?"

When I returned home, I talked to Peter again on the phone. "Yes, I've heard – such a shame. Connelly was hurt but will survive…Jackie is ok," Peter said. "I'm coming home now. I love you."

"I love you too, Darling," I said.

The funeral lasted three days after the assassination. Peter and I watched the wake at the Rotunda on television. On the third day, Jacqueline Kennedy along with family members led the funeral procession. Behind was "Black Jack," the riderless black horse, wearing a saddle and bridle with boots in the stirrups facing backwards. A team of horses pulled the caisson, a sign of a fallen hero, carrying Kennedy's body from the White House to the Cathedral of St. Matthews. Most impressive was "Little John John" saluting his father's casket.

John F. Kennedy was buried in Arlington National Cemetery, his plot lit by an Eternal Flame.

To this day, there is speculation as to who assassinated John F. Kennedy…was it Lee Harvey Oswald acting alone or was it a conspiracy?

Barbara Engler, a poet and close friend of mine, wrote the following poem in Junior High at age 15. Like Barbara, hundreds of thousands were affected by the death of Kennedy:

"November 1963"

"The shots rang out!
A volley of three
Kennedy and Connelly
At first the people
Could not heed
The horror of
That monstrous deed.

A short swearing in
Aboard Air Force One
New President Lyndon Johnson
Jackie in her bloodied suit
Bares witness to
The death of Camelot.

The caisson,
Pulled by a team of 6
Bore the coffin
Past history's witnesses
A Riderless horse
Boots reversed in the stirrups
To face the back."

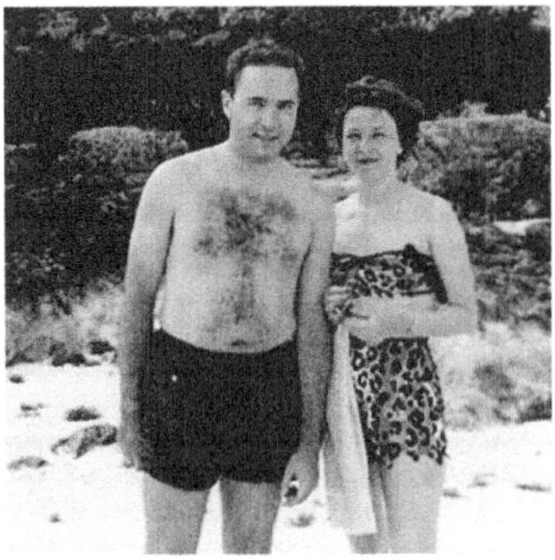

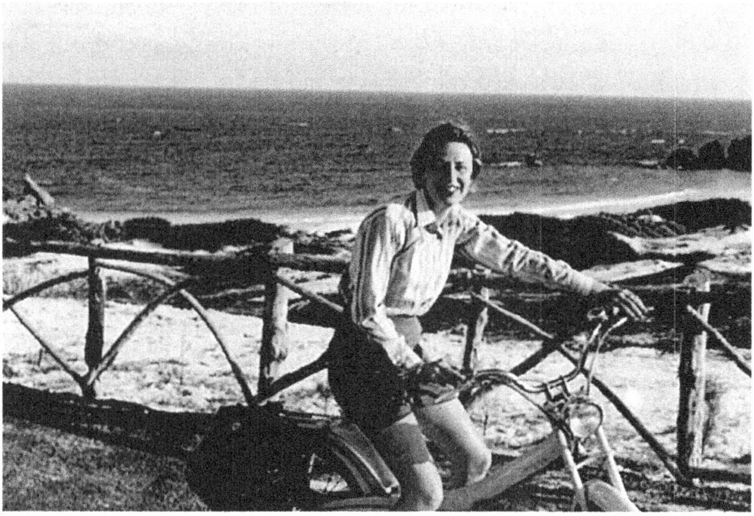

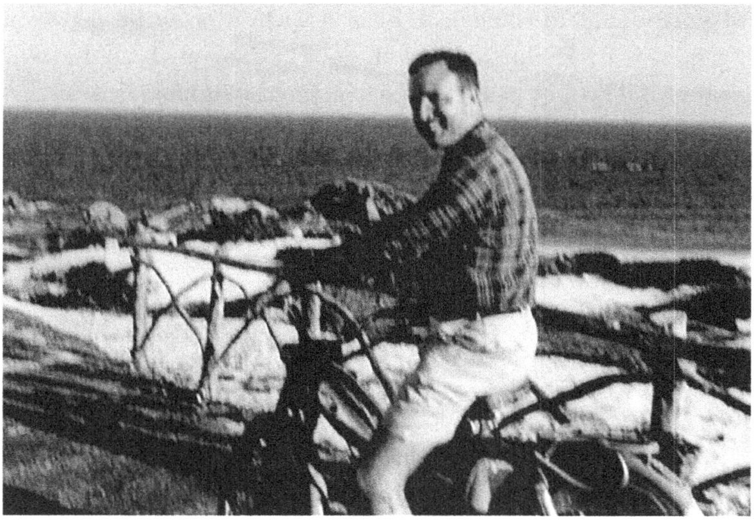

# Love Letters from India

On January 22, 1964, I sent off Peter and Dale Gooden, an Engineer, at John F. Kennedy Airport. They were again headed for India via Istanbul. We checked the baggage and had a few minutes to talk. Dale headed for the gate.

"Don't forget to write," I said handing him a love note which he put in his coat pocket…"read it on the plane."

"Sweet-Love, I hate to leave you." He kissed me on the lips. "That will have to last a long time!"

"I know…it's all right…just hurry home. Remember I'm in your pocket!" He gave me a long, gentle hug. "I love, love, love you, Sweetheart," I whispered in his ear.

"I love you more," he laughed and squeezed my hand.

The BOAC plane began to board. Dale called out, "Thanks, Ceci, keep in touch with Judy." I nodded smiling, and threw Peter a kiss.

Looking out the airport's bay window, I hoped that Peter might get a glimpse of me. The plane taxied down the runway and out of sight.

I had gotten into the Vauxhall when a BOAC plane flew low overhead. "Have a safe trip, my Darling," I said out loud. I hung my head down upon the steering wheel and became bathed in tears. I would miss him terribly!

Peter and I were passionately and deeply in love. We knew we could get through anything as long as we had each other. Writing love letters was even more important now. They would keep us close. As it turned out, his stay lasted almost three months. The trip was trying for us; nevertheless, we found that our love continued to grow amazingly stronger.

I quote excerpts from Peter's letters. Not only are they loving and charming but descriptive of his surroundings:

January 23, 1964
"Istanbul Hilton
Istanbul, Turkey

My Darling:

We arrived here safely last night after a trip which was delayed several hours by fog which prevented us from landing at London

Airport, forcing us to land at Gatwick Airport outside of London and wait for several hours.

Your wonderful letter really warmed the cockles of my heart and made my tummy reach out to you (what a lot of action to be caused by a letter!).

Take care of my Sweetie-poose.

I love you,

Peter"

January 27, 1964
"ASHOKA HOTEL
NEW DELHI

My Darling:

Thank you so much for your letters of the 22nd and 23rd. I have just mailed the letter which I dashed off to you a few minutes ago, and hope it reaches you before this, just to create the illusion of a little extra mail.

Dale and I had a good sleep Wednesday night, then hired a car Thursday for a three hour drive around Istanbul. The city looks much like other western European cities. The most marked differences being the fact that almost everywhere you look you see Moslem mosques, with their domes and towers. Our guide took us inside one of them, the "Blue Mosque," while the faithful were at prayer (apparently nobody objects to this sort of thing).

The weather in Istanbul was the worst they'd had in years, and it was snowing when we left on Thursday evening. When we arrived in New Delhi Friday morning we found that the city has been undergoing an unusually cold spell – overcoat weather.

Sunday morning we watched the Republic Day parade, which consisted of troops, tanks, cavalry, troops mounted on camels, elephants carrying people playing musical instruments, in addition to just about every civic group in New Delhi. The parade concluded with a "flypast" by jet planes at low altitude. We sat in temporary grandstands which, combined with the cold weather, gave the affair some of the aura of a football game.

I miss you my little sweet Darling, and keep dreaming about you. How about that!

I love you,

Peter"

February13, 1964

Thursday

"Mrs. Peter T. Hitchcock

133 West 12th Street

New York 11, N.Y.

U.S.A.

My dearest, most wonderful Husband:

Judy just called from the airport to say that she is on her way – she, and I, can't believe it. Am most happy for her as she has wanted to go to Italy for years, as you know. I'll miss her as we have talked each day to compare notes. I wish so that I can be on my way also but really you can't imagine what fun I am having fixing up the apartment. There is so much to do! Oh, Darling, you'll be so proud of our home.

As yet, I haven't heard from you for three days. Dale's letter from Judy yesterday said that you were working from 9 am until 11 pm every day. Am afraid you are working too hard. The way things are going, it looks as though you might spend the month of March also. Oh, Darling, I hope not. It will be four weeks this coming Tuesday. I really have counted on a good seven weeks though which will take you to the first week of March. Well, I have enough to keep me busy here with our apartment.

Next week I want to do a little painting, especially the kitchen which the Smiths didn't have done. I thought I could do it anyway. As you can see, I am busy – but still very lonely. I miss and need you so badly and oh, do I ever love my Darling-Love. Take care of my Sweetie-Man.

I love you,

Ceci

P. S. I wish so that you were here – I could almost eat you up – not quite, but I would like to be in your arms. I love you."

February 14, 1964
"Mrs. Peter T. Hitchcock
133 West 12th Street
New York 11, N.Y.
U.S.A.

FOR THE 7,634,821st TIME........I Love You.
Yes please!
Happy Valentine's Day, my Darling.
Your Spoose loves you very, very, very much.
Ceci"

February 22, 1964
"ASHOKA HOTEL
NEW DELHI

My most-loved Sweetie-spoose (how about that!):

This last week has been extremely hectic, with conferences going on endlessly, it would seem. The word "conferences" includes a lot of almost never-ending arguments with Bhanu, but that certainly should be no surprise to you.

At any rate, I worry because I haven't written to you during the past few days – knowing how much I depend on receiving your letters, I hope that I haven't made you wonder what's going on.

At any rate, as we've both noticed, writing to one another really does give us a vital link between us. The act of writing to you, of feeling that we're talking together really helps to get rid of the depression which I've begun to feel as a result of being away from you

Needless to say, Sweet-Darling, I miss you more and more every day. I keep constantly thinking about you, what a beautiful, sweet and sagacious little Spoose you are! Even though the weather is nice in New Delhi right now, I would so much rather be in cold, wet, rainy New York, with a nice fire to keep my Darling warm while you move around our apartment, look at TV, iron, or whatever.

Also, thank you for your two letters from Princeton last weekend, plus your letters of last Monday and Tuesday. How I wish I could have you in my pocket (or bed – naughty?)

Take care, my Love, and I'll be able to write much more from now on.

I love you,
Peter"

February 25, 1964
"ASHOKA HOTEL
NEW DELHI

My Darling:

Just a quick note so that I can get this into the mail along with some other things which I'm taking downtown to the post office in hopes of getting them onto one of the flights taking off this evening.

Bhanu will probably arrive tonight, which means more tiresome arguments over every Goddamn detail which anybody can think up. If, at some (hopefully remote) time you may consider me to be temporarily surly, just console yourself with the thought that you're not married to Bhanu. There, thanks for listening to my momentary bitching!

The weather is getting quite warm now, which is some consolation. Within another month it should be back up to the 100's temperatures. Needless to say, I hope to have someone write to me from New Delhi to let me know just how Goddamn hot it is.

Looking out from Dale's balcony a few minutes ago I saw a bunch of off-duty BOAC or Quantas pilots, hostesses, etc. relaxing on beach chairs in the sun. Sometimes the sight makes me think how nice it must be to be young and carefree again, without worries which you have to live and contend with constantly. (Things are not that bad, though).

Incidentally, you certainly are a key figure in our communications set-up, or so it would appear. Dale learns about Judy and I learn about Allied through you. I guess whatever Larry finds out depends on what you decide to tell Kathy.

In all seriousness, though, I wish you'd check with Mary Smith next Monday afternoon to see whether John has received a report from me dated the 24th and mailed at Palam Airport today. The reason I'm concerned is that this is a letter with a number of stamps on it. A similar letter from Dale to Norm apparently was not received (we found out, of course, because we referred to it in other memos). Apparently, if you don't watch them cancel the stamps, post office employees sometimes steam them off for resale. The letter just doesn't get there. I've always watched them stamp and endorse the envelopes because I wanted to make sure they got into the appropriate box for U.S. delivery. Now I'll be doubly careful.

Every day I seem to miss you more. Dreamed about you last night, yes please!

I love you,

Peter

P.S. – The torn edges are due to the fact that the pages got caught in my briefcase. Don't blame the Indian post office.

Peter"

February 29, 1964

"ASHOKA HOTEL

NEW DELHI

My Darling:

Thank you for your letters of the 22nd and 24th. They really helped to bring you closer to me, and were great morale boosters. I'm so proud of you for the great job you've been doing painting our apartment.

For some reason I keep thinking back to the wonderful time we had together in Bermuda last year, and keep picturing you in my mind. It made me feel so good to see such a happy and relaxed loved-spoose. Even looking at a picture of the lakes in Kashmir makes me think of you and Bermuda, because there were several pictures in a book which I read while we were at the Coral Beach Club.

I hate this separation more and more. Take care of my Sweetie-Spoose.

I love you,

Peter"

March 1, 1964
"ASHOKA HOTEL
NEW DELHI

My Darling:

This is the second letter I will have written to you today, but probably will get to you before the morning one, inasmuch as that one has been mailed in the Ashoka mail system, while I probably will take this one out to Palam Airport to mail it tomorrow, along with a memo for John G. It usually saves a day or so kicking around in the New Delhi post office.

I have been working away today in my room with an hour off to lie in the sun and try to start a tan. My other big activity today has been missing you, my little sweetie-love. I can picture very clearly how lovely you looked the night you saw us off. You know, I really liked that hairdo, and hope that you can keep that lovely effect. You'd be a beauty spoose anyway, of course!

Our time element is still uncertain, but it looks as though we'll be stuck here for several weeks.

I really hate to seem business-like as this letter looks. I love and miss you so much, my little cutie-sweetie! Look after my love.

I love you,
Peter"

March 11, 1964
"ASHOKA HOTEL
NEW DELHI

My Sweet-Darling:

Right now I still favor taking you on that European trip, particularly since it is really getting hot now – like New York in late June or early July, and getting hotter every day.

Even having gone through this before, I never realized that I could miss my Little Darling Wife so much. I love you Sweetie!

Peter"

March 18, 1964
Wednesday
"ASHOKA HOTEL
NEW DELHI

My Darling:

As the days go by I keep missing you more and more, but I guess that really isn't anything in the way of news. The one consolation is that I've been able to concoct the nicest series of daydreams about us...yes please, but I do have to keep putting such thoughts out of my mind. I always let them stay for a little while, though!

Your wonderful letters of the 11th and 13th both arrived Monday. That's pretty darn good for the mail service at both ends. Your letter of the 13th said that you almost called me "the other night". Perhaps that was Thursday night. The reason I mention it is that I was so depressed from missing you that I almost called you, just to say I love you. Great minds think alike. The trouble is that once the call got through we might only hear an occasional word which we spoke to one another, which would be terribly frustrating. It might be confusing as well, since you might think that the incomprehensible words and static represented an attempt to tell you something about our plans. Anyway, it still is a tempting thought.

The only way poor Dale can learn of where Judy is (or was) is through you. He's somewhat unhappy that she doesn't keep him informed at all as to where she is or is going. He's trying to reach her, hopefully in Rome, but will probably have to tell her to go on home.

We're still trying to get at least a few basic items from the Government, but it's a slow matter, dealing with an almost incredibly ponderous bureaucracy.

Take care of my Darling
Peter"

March 21, 1964
"Mrs. Peter T. Hitchcock
133 West 12th Street
New York 11, New York
U.S.A.

My Darling:

I will be spending Easter here (Princeton) as we spent Thanksgiving in Bronxville. How I wish you could be here.

Goodness, do I miss you! How I yearn for your arms, to hear your voice, and to start living a normal life of cooking for my Husband and taking care of him. But pretty soon, I keep telling myself.

Take good care of yourself. I want to get this into the mail so will close for now. I love you, my Darling, and needless to say I miss you terribly.

Ceci"

*****

Two incidences occurred while Peter was in India. I would tell Peter about them when he returned.

Early one evening at the apartment Phillip Morehouse called. He was in the City on business.

"Lee, how are you?" he asked enthusiastically.

"Well, how are you?" I answered back recognizing his voice.

"I had to call your mother to get your phone number. Can we meet tonight, sometime?" he asked. I laughed.

"You know, Phillip, I'm married now." There was silence on the phone.

"How is Peter doing?" he inquired.

"He's in India on business for Allied. I hope to join him in Frankfurt, Germany, shortly. How's your job going?" I questioned.

"Please won't you meet me?" he begged. I was becoming impatient. "Phillip, I'm a married woman," I repeated. I've never been so happy in love. Why don't you try marriage? It's wonderful. Listen…I'm expecting an important call. I have to go." What a white lie, I laughed to myself!

"O.K.…I'll call you again soon when I'm back in town," he sighed and hung up.

"You'll be wasting your time!" I uttered out loud. Suddenly I felt a letter coming on. I would write Peter.

The other incident happened in my office at NYU. At the end of the day, an associate came over to my desk. "Hi, Sean," I said. "What can I do for you?"

"How would you like to go out for a cocktail now?" he asked smiling, as he leaned on my desk. He had probably learned through office gossip that Peter was in India.

"I'm flattered…You're kidding, of course," I answered quite taken back. "You know we're both married…besides, I wouldn't do that behind Peter's back."

"Well...if you change your mind, you know where to find me," he balked smugly and returned to his office. I was both flabbergasted and mystified as his wife was charming and ever so attractive.

"Peter...Peter," I pleaded to myself as I got up from my desk. "Please...please come home soon!" I put my coat on, said "goodnight" to those around me, and headed home.

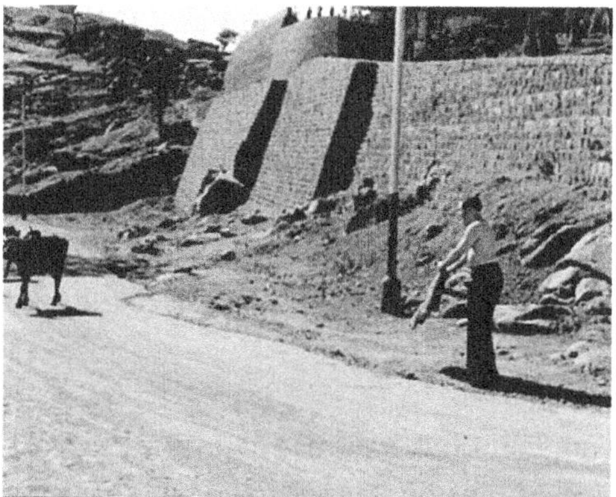

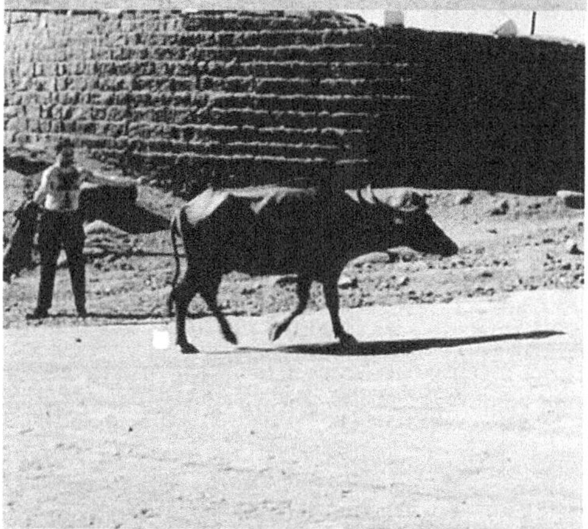

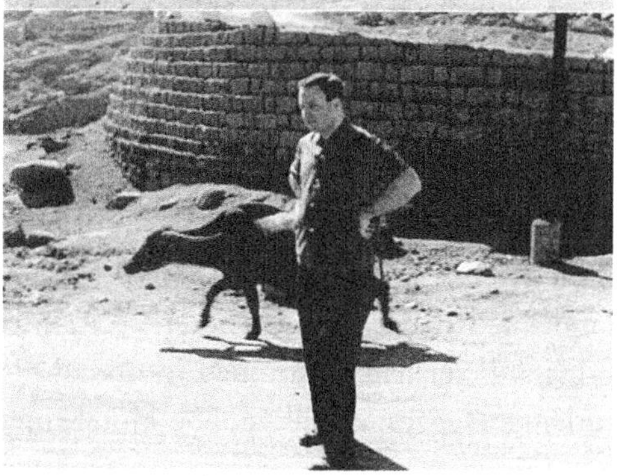

# Joining Peter in Europe

At last Peter's Western Union Telegrams, dated March 22nd and 23rd, arrived stating that he wanted me to join him. He and Dale would be leaving India for Frankfurt, Germany, on the 26th. That meant I would meet him on the 27th giving me only four days to prepare. Thankfully, I was able to book a seat on PanAm's flight 72 nonstop to Frankfurt. It was a blessing that Dorothy McDonald okayed the trip for the two-week vacation, giving me the day off before I was to leave. I was glad I had had the foresight to purchase American Express traveler checks and the necessary cash I needed, as Peter had asked. In one of Peter's past letters he suggested I bring warm clothes, mix and match, a heavy wool sweater and coat. Because I had to work during the day, I used lunch hours and evenings to accomplish all that I needed to do. I sent Peter the following RCA Cablegram:

> "Arriving Frankfurt Saturday Morning 9:15.
> PanAm 72 Nonstop. Have a good trip.
> Love my Darling.Ceci"

Luckily, I had purchased large and small, zippered, red plaid suitcases and a carryon to match the weekend before; however, I was frantic to find padlocks small enough for the luggage. After several hours trying different hardware stores in the Village, I finally found what I needed.

I'll never forget the long, seemingly endless, nine-hour trip to Frankfurt. I especially remember sitting in an aisle seat next to a grimy, unhygienic, uncombed, bearded guy who sipped vodka from a pint bottle throughout the whole trip. I pretended to sleep most of the time but was ready to complain to the flight attendant at any moment.

I couldn't believe I was meeting my Sweetheart after such a lengthy separation of almost three months.

When we arrived at the Frankfurt Airport which was on time, I hurriedly left the plane...but there was no Peter! I proceeded to Customer Service, holding tightly my petite German dictionary. Luckily, I found someone who could speak English and told him my dilemma. I was told my luggage had not been put on the plane but would be delivered to the hotel...but there was no Americana Hotel. Thank goodness, Peter had mentioned in one of his letters the hotel was new. The kind gentleman suggested calling The Hotel InterContinental to see if a Peter Hitchcock had checked in. Indeed, all of this was nerve-racking to me. I was scared.

Yes, Peter was at The Hotel InterContinental but why hadn't he met me? Obviously, we had no cell phones in those days and couldn't communicate with each other! I was assured by Customer Service that my luggage would be delivered to the hotel room around two am in the morning. I wondered...what else could go wrong after a horrible plane ride, no husband, no luggage, and wrong hotel! I was shaking, apprehensive and ready to scream. I got ahold of myself, flagged a cab, and headed to the Hotel InterContinental. I must have given the cab driver too much money as he was absolutely overjoyed, thanking me several times. I didn't care. I just wanted to find Peter!

I went to the front desk of the hotel asking if a Peter Hitchcock had checked in. Indeed he had. I was given a room key and took the elevator up to our floor. Our room was at the end of a long hall. Upon opening the door, I found a very sick husband fast asleep. The bathroom floor was covered with vomit and blood. "Great!" I thought.

"My sweet Darling-Love," I whispered in his ear. What in the world has happened to you?" I kissed him on his warm perspiring forehead. He opened his sluggish hazel eyes and gave me the biggest smile. "I think you have a fever."

"Sweet-Love, am I glad to see you! I'm sorry I couldn't meet you. I must have a touch of the flu or ate something on the plane that disagreed with me. Don't worry."

"Don't worry!" I exclaimed. "There's blood and vomit all over the bathroom floor." Before he could say anything, I grabbed the phone and put in a call to the hotel's house doctor. Thankfully, he was able to come immediately. Upon learning that Peter had been in the Navy, he wanted to put him in the naval hospital.

"No...no," I said. "I'm sure he is physically rundown as he has just returned from India after a three month business stay. Can't you give him an antibiotic, aspirin to lower his temperature, and something for his queasiness?"

"My wife went to nursing school in the States," Peter laughed. "I just need rest." The doctor agreed and said he would be around tomorrow if I needed him. "However, you'll have to find a pharmacy. The front desk can help you." I thanked him, walking him to the door, and called Housekeeping to clean up the bathroom.

"Sweetheart, I'll be back. Get some sleep," I said and nervously hurried down to the front desk. I was told the pharmacy was up the street at the light on the corner.

I was successful in finding the pharmacy and, with the help of my petite German dictionary and the little I remembered from a course I had taken at St. Mary's, was able to fill the prescriptions and purchase aspirin. At least something was going right!

That night and the next day, Easter Sunday, I used room service. Peter ate and slept. For me, I must say bed felt good. However, I was awakened, as promised, with a knock on the door at two am. I was glad to see the bellboy with my luggage. I gave him a tip, closed the door, and crawled back into bed. I hadn't slept a wink on the plane!

On Easter, with the help of medications, food and sleep, Peter began to bounce back. I too caught up on sleep!

The following card I had purchased in New York City:

> "To my Husband at Easter: Happy Easter, Mr. Wonderful, and happy springtime, too, from your loving Mrs. Lucky, who thinks the world of you!" To my Darling, my wonderful Sweetie-Man. A very Happy Easter. I love you,
> Ceci"
>
> "P.S. When I bought this I certainly didn't think that I would be giving this to you in person!"

Thankfully, even though he wasn't feeling up to par, Peter joined Dale Gooden and kept the appointment with Lurgi Monday morning. I, in the meantime, took advantage of the time by reading up on Frankfurt. I especially was interested in the barge ride down the Rhein River and suggested it to Peter when he returned in time for lunch, which we had at the hotel's café. He agreed as he had wanted to show me Frankfurt's beautiful countryside. He was sure the deal with India would go through. We had one day to take the boat ride and then we would have to head to Berlin for two days.

While Peter rested, I adventured outside to a jeweler which was conveniently located next to the pharmacy to purchase a stein charm to add onto the bracelet that my Grandmother Myers had given me from Switzerland. It was Peter's idea!

Early Tuesday morning we took the relaxing day trip by barge downstream, or north, on the Rhein River which was some 820 miles long...Germany's busiest river. I stood in awe as we passed the mountain-like countryside remarkably lush and grassy green. Clay or dirt roads zigzagged through vast vineyards that crisscrossed each other. Next to them were parceled fields on the hilly terrain divided, I believe, by stone walls or wooden fences. Quaint winemaking villages and charming small towns dotted the colorful landscape along the water's edge. Above the steep rocky crags were romantic, fairylike, stone castles and ancient ruins. It was all amazingly beautiful and unforgettable!

Peter and I wanted to travel as far as Cologne but we ran out of time. We got off at Dusseldorf and returned to Frankfurt to prepare for our trip to Berlin.

Back at the Hotel InterContinental Peter received a phone call from Dale Gooden saying he wasn't feeling well and would stay in Frankfurt. Judy would probably go to Paris for a few days. They would join us in Brussels, Belgium.

*****

I quote from a letter to my parents written from the Berlin Hilton on April 5, 1964:

> "Dearest Mother and Mike:
>
> We had a very pleasant trip yesterday morning arriving by plane around twelve-thirty. As you can see, we are staying at the Berlin Hilton Hotel. Reservations are so hard to get both here and Amsterdam at this time of year that we had to take what was offered us.
>
> After lunch yesterday we took the four hour bus tour of East and West Berlin. What an experience and my how depressing. As we entered "Checkpoint Charlie" no photo-taking was allowed. Both East and West soldiers were on either side of the wall. Once we got into the Eastern Sector we had to have our passports examined. One soldier even examined the underside of the bus (in case someone was trying to get in). The streets were absolutely bare and if any people, no smiles. What a depressing sight. The other depressing part of East Berlin is the utter ruin of their buildings. They haven't been touched since the bombing of the 2nd World War! Of course, only the government buildings have been renovated and a few apartment buildings also.
>
> The wall itself is 30 miles long. Most of it is so high that one can't look on the other side. Where it is low enough to see across, the E. Germans have put sheets of cardboard about 1000 feet from the wall – to keep a West Berliner from seeing an East Berliner. Of course, there is a triple layer of wire on top of the wall, and to make it easier to locate one who might be trying to escape at night the East Berlin side of the wall has been painted white! We were shown the

various places where East Berliners tried to escape either to their deaths or to their freedom. A sad scene was the wall around the cemetery and church (which was well populated before the wall was built). Unable to get into the cemetery, people here hooked wreaths on the wall at Christmas time. They are still there! The church and the rector's house (beautiful red brick) are not being used and haven't since the wall was built. Believe-it-or-not, where the East Berliners did not put wire on top of the wall they put broken glass laid in cement!! – just horrible.

At the point of returning to the Western side our guides changed as they did before we entered E. Berlin. We were told that around 4 o'clock there was a lot of firing of guns on the E. Berlin side, probably someone trying to escape! It all is unbelievable. (Also, we saw a young man standing on a roof of a store waving to a loved one, probably in E. Berlin).

We will probably take a walk around the hotel this afternoon. Berlin is so big – fourth biggest city in size in the world so we were told.

Love to you both,
Ceci"

In the above letter to my parents I neglected to mention that we were allowed to leave the bus in East Berlin to wander around the ruins. For some reason a soldier spotted Peter and watched him closely...probably thinking he could be a spy. He followed us wherever we went. I suggested that we return to the bus where our passports were examined. Peter mentioned that he experienced the same kind of treatment when he was in the Korean War! We were happy to return to "Checkpoint Charlie". It was quite unsettling. Peter remarked, "It reminded me of my days in the Navy...the same kind of suspicion."

We left Berlin via Hamburg arriving in Amsterdam, Holland, the largest city and Dutch capital of the Netherlands. Staying at the Amsterdam Hilton, we had just three days. Peter, having been there before, decided a good way for me to see the City was to take a boat ride on the canals the next morning. Our tour guide told us that Amsterdam has about 100 kilometers of canals, 90 islands, and 1500 bridges forming a canal ring belt around the City. Alongside the main canals are about 1550 majestic towering buildings...some on tree-lined streets with parked cars and bikes.

Later, we enjoyed walking past the various stores except for the jeweler. Peter suggested we purchase a charm for my 18 karat gold bracelet – a windmill. He was always so thoughtful and wanted to make me happy and, of course, vice versa! From there, we passed the "Red-light district"- a group of storefronts or cubicles each housing a woman, who was either walking back and forth or sitting and waiting at her large window for a client. We were being watched closely as we passed by. "I'm glad I'm not one of them!" I whispered to Peter. He laughed with a broad smile. "I'm glad you're not the type, Sweet-Love!"

We returned to the Amsterdam Hilton for dinner and signed up for a car rental to explore the Hague the next day. Leaving early that morning after a hearty breakfast, we picked up our convertible Ford Mustang and headed north on the causeway. We could have taken a bike tour but we wanted to be independent. We passed quaint villages along the dikes, deep valleys of water with stone banks. There were picturesque and graceful windmills of different sizes, turned by electric pumps, scattered on farms with divided fields of different colored seas of tulips. As we reached the northern tip, we had to turn around. We parked and, for a moment, were in awe of the North Sea and scenic countryside. I took a picture with our 35 mm camera of Peter sitting behind the wheel of the convertible. Climbing back into the car, I kissed him on the cheek. "Isn't the countryside breathtaking?" I asked, staring into his sparkling hazel eyes. "I love you, Darling. I'm glad we did this!" Peter gave me a hug. "I love you too," he whispered. He started the car engine to return to the city. "Yes please!" I said smiling. I marveled on how close we were...a strong chemistry that bonded us together. We were forever in love.

On April 10$^{th}$ we continued our European trip staying at the Hotel Metropole where we met Dale Gooden, Judy, and an associate with his wife for a business dinner at the hotel that evening. The next day the three men met again discussing India. All agreed the project would go through. We saw little of French speaking Brussels, Capital of Belgium, well known for its beer and chocolates – only the downtown- "the Grand Place," or town square, where people gathered and meandered. Cafes and stores were in stunning Gothic styled buildings that surrounded the plaza.

Peter, fluent in French, bought another gold charm – a government building- for my bracelet.

After having lunch with the Goodens in one of the cafes, we headed for the airport which would take us to London, England. Peter could now put business behind him...a trip we were really looking forward to, as he had lived there in the Navy for two years.

We arrived at Heathrow Airport in London, the capital city of England. Checking in at the Cumberland Hotel on Oxford Street and Park Lane, our room overlooked the beautiful, lush Hyde Park, one of many parks in London. We loved the hotel, and especially enjoyed the extra soft, cozy double sized bed with its large feathery down quilt. It felt good as we were tired from all the traveling!

We took advantage of the short time we had before returning to the States. Peter rented a car which proved to be a good way to sightsee. He took me to familiar places he enjoyed while in the Navy, having no problem driving on the left side of the road with the steering wheel on the right side of the car. We visited the western part of London in main downtown namely bustling Piccadilly Circus, with its many cars, double-decker buses, taxis, and trucks surrounded by restaurants, cafes, and stores galore. I remember seeing a bobby directing traffic.

We then came to the well-known, enormous Trafalgar Square, parked, and walked to its center to the water fountain which was surrounded by a stone wall where people enjoyed sitting. There were, of course, tour buses, street performers, people gathered taking pictures and feeding hungry pigeons that flitted up and down in flocks or individually racing for a bite. In the distance, we could see the net of bridges...on the Thames River...the Tower Bridge, which took eight years to build, and London Bridge. Then there was the Pool, where tall ships, cruise liners, and steamers could pass through. After lunch, we shopped at the seven story Harrods, a luxurious department store with its many escalators. Peter brought me a gold Queen's crown for my bracelet. We also bought silk Liberty ties and scarves, as Christmas wasn't too far away.

Two days before we were to leave London, we took a double-decker bus to Buckingham Palace to see the Changing of the Guard...a tradition of marching military soldiers in red, black, and gold uniforms changing posts. The soldiers are there to protect the Royals. Watching the guards march in formation was fascinating, precise, and yet extremely beautiful...but not a smile on any face! We were lucky that day as the military band marched past us and up the street, a picture-perfect scene.

On our last day, Peter took me to his apartment, where he lived while in the Navy. His was on the corner of the first floor of the six-story modern, white building. "It looks like they're tearing it down," he commented peeking through a window of the empty apartment. There was construction debris all around.

"How sad! That's where you learned how to make gravy and Poule a la Hitchcock," I joked. Peter laughed. "I really enjoyed living there. Am glad I got a glimpse of it before demolition." I know he felt sad but we took pictures which

Peter was happy to have. Later, we found out that a Hilton Hotel had been built in its place!

We were sorry to leave London but happy to return to our cozy, garden apartment in New York City. It was perfect timing as Peter developed a rash – itchy pustules, under each armpit. He first noticed a few in Frankfurt. Perhaps that is why he felt lousy and lacked energy.

We saw Dr. Edlich, our primary doctor, the next day. He said he had never seen a rash like that before; however, he felt it was a virus Peter had contracted from the Ashoka's swimming pool! He told Peter to stay home for a few days, rest, and try 100% Hydrocortisone Cream. As for me, I returned to work at NYU.

Happily, the rash disappeared in two weeks. Since Peter had five weeks' vacation, his boss, John G., suggested he take a week off which we did by returning to Bermuda. We thoroughly enjoyed ourselves in spite of the Red Tide, an algae that kept us from swimming. It was the best advice we had received as Peter was a new person when we returned to the City.

The rest of 1964 seemed to fly by. Thankfully, Peter never returned to India after the three months' stay. Instead, the Indians came to Peter in New York City! One night we had to entertain Bhanu. We took him to an Indian restaurant. Peter was glad I could share this experience with him instead of his doing it alone. We enjoyed the relaxed evening, but I must say the Chicken Tandoori was a bit biting for me...but not for Bhanu who poured a hearty helping of hot sauce over the meat. I laughed remarking, "How can you stand so much hot sauce?" His reply was, "Indian food isn't Indian unless you have hot sauce and lots of curry!"

Peter was proud of me that night and commented that he wished I had been with him during the negotiations in India. "You are a sagacious spoose," he frequently told me.

In August, we went sailing with Edie and Alan in Bayville, Long Island one weekend. What a perfectly fun time we had. And, of course, Alan and Peter did a bit of fishing for Saturday night's dinner.

Then onto the World's Fair of 1964 in Montreal, Canada...we enjoyed the overnight sleeper more than the Expo itself! Both of us have traveled extensively by Pullman...I at St. Mary's during the three years I was there, going back and forth from Raleigh, North Carolina to Princeton via Trenton, New Jersey...and Peter from Exeter, New Hampshire to Bronxville, New York and during his travels. He'd find any excuse to use the train!

Going to Montreal our Pullman suite was small and cozy with a bathroom. We left after dinner on a Friday arriving early that next morning. The ride was fairly smooth but bumpy when cars were being changed in the middle of the night. We awakened. Peter's arm was on my waist as I slept on my side facing him. "I love you, Darling," he whispered kissing me on the lips. "I'm so glad I married you." "My Sweet-Darling," I said smiling, half asleep. "I adore you, too." "How about that," he answered. "Come here!" He took me into his arms and, before I knew it, we entered into the world of Inanity.

Being with Peter gave me such peace and security. I marveled at how happy we were, enjoying each other in every way and having fun. Peter always put me first making sure I was thoroughly loved and cuddled. It was his way of showing me he loved me.

We had breakfast in the Diner, a fun experience…eating on a train. The World's Fair was outside of Montreal; thus, we took a bus which took us to the Fair. There, we decided to take the tram in spite of the fact we both had a fear of heights! The trip gave us a birds-eye view of the Fair grounds. We then walked our feet off visiting many pavilions, especially India, the Republic of China, the Caribbean, and Bell Telephone. Tired, we finally took the train from one pavilion to another. But leave it up to me to do something crazy…getting off the train during one stop, I left my purse on the car seat…too late…off the train went! I yelled at the attendant frantically, who in turn got in touch with the attendant by walkie-talkie ahead of us. He had the purse and would give it to Lost and Found. "You are a very lucky lady!" the young man called out. With directions in hand we had no trouble finding the Lost and Found and retrieving the purse; needless to say, we were most relieved as I had a fair amount of cash Peter had given me. We were indeed lucky!

Later that afternoon we went into Montreal, a beautiful city, for a bite to eat at a French restaurant. We then boarded the train back to New York City.

In early November Edie and Alan invited us to the Army-Navy game in Philadelphia, Pennsylvania. It is a college rivalry game between the Army Black Knights (the United States Military Academy in West Point, New York) and the Navy Midshipmen (the United States Naval Academy in Annapolis, Maryland). Navy won. Needless to say, Peter was extremely happy. To me, the game was exciting no matter who had the ball. We took lots of pictures, especially at half-time, of the marching bands and their formations.

After returning home by train, we decided to take the subway to Greenwich Village. Little did we know we were being followed by two grubby punks, as Peter called them. Edie and Alan had climbed the stairs to the upper platform. Eyeing the two men, I nudged Peter and shouted, "Hey, Alan, wait for us." Thankfully, the boys ran off as we hurried up the stairs. Both of us were shaken and never forgot the incident. I guess we were overdressed for the Village, as

Peter wore a long camel hair coat and scarf, and I in my purple wool coat with the fur collar. We learned a lesson to always be aware of our surroundings.

*****

By now I was working part-time at NYU which gave me more time to be with Peter on weekends. This was short-lived as Peter called me at the office early one morning several weeks later, around November 17th. "Darling, Mommy is sick. Her doctor wants to put her in the hospital."

"Call him back...tell him we're on our way. What's the next train to Bronxville?" I asked.

"It leaves at eleven am. I'll meet you at Grand Central Station," he said. "I love you."

"And I'll go to the apartment to pack a few things for us. I'd better dash. I love you, too," I said hurriedly. I explained the situation to Dorothy McDonald, who was most understanding, and walked to the apartment.

Peter and I barely made the train. Upon arrival in Bronxville, we picked up the Vauxhall at the garage and drove to Avon Road. There, an ambulance was parked in front of the house. We found Elinor on a stretcher in the hallway entrance. She took my hand. "The house is yours to clean out," she said. "Take good care of Inky. "I will," I promised, reassuring her. "We'll follow you to the hospital." Peter's sister, Anne, was at the house, and Gaylord came down from Dartmouth. I was glad to have them around as they would relieve Peter at the Lawrence Hospital.

Five days later Elinor died from cirrhosis of the liver. The funeral was held at Christ Church. We were amazed at the number of Bronxville friends she had that attended the service.

When Peter and I were finally alone at the house, we hugged. "I'm sorry, Sweetheart. She was a wonderful lady," I said. "We will miss her." Peter had tears in his eyes. "It's o.k. ...let it out," I continued, kissing him on the cheek.

"You know what this means," he said emphatically wiping the tears away. "We have to move!" I felt extremely sad, too. I hated to leave the City, but we had no other choice.

"We'll be o.k., Sweetheart, as long as we have each other. We'll get through this!" In a way we were lucky to be moving into such a beautiful house...our first real home.

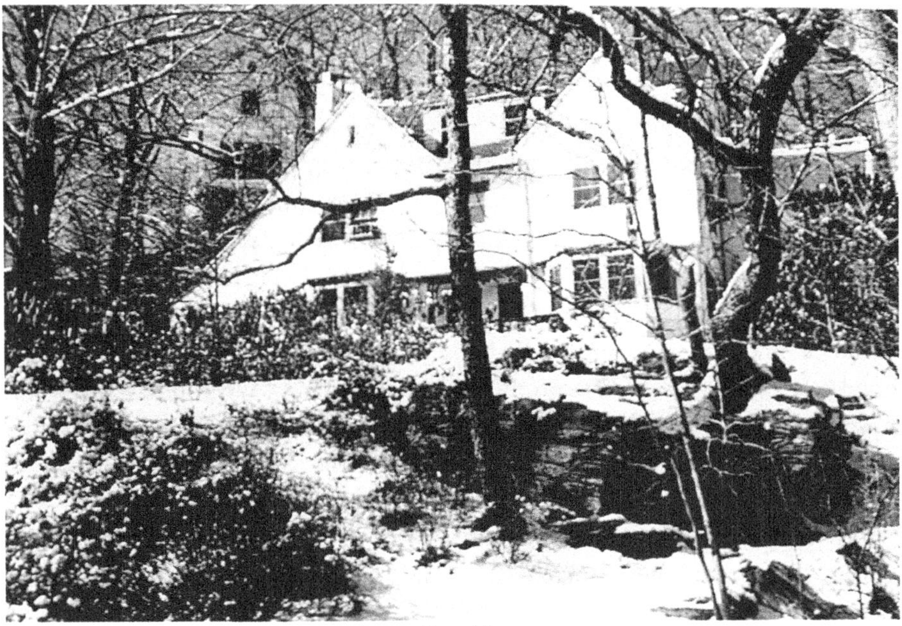

Avon Road house

# Part Four: Life Challenges

## Moving to Bronxville

Peter wanted me to leave my NYU job. It wouldn't be cost-effective for both of us to commute every day to the City from Bronxville, New York. I, therefore, gave notice, which enabled me to prepare for the move, while Peter continued to work at Allied Chemical. Luckily, the apartment came furnished, meaning we had only our personal belongings to pack. We were certainly sad to leave our cozy apartment and City life. I must admit, also, that I was somewhat apprehensive as Peter's two sisters, Anne and Kathy, would be living with us. Anne and I were good friends, but Kathy was unstable and mentally ill, diagnosed with Schizophrenia. At times she was difficult, out of control and unbearable to have around. Kathy was extremely bright, an Emma Willard School and a Columbia University graduate. Peter said that at the age of eight she jumped off of a beanbag hammock and landed on her head. At one time she entered Stamford Hall, Stamford, Connecticut…a rehabilitation hospital. Ironically, that's where the ambulance took my alcoholic father in a strait jacket.

Kathy married a medical school graduate from a prominent family in Bronxville. She was caught cheating on him, which he witnessed. As a result, he divorced her…this all happened during Peter's third year at Columbia Law School when we were dating. She interrupted many an evening at the apartment with long tiresome phone conversations. I suggested he not talk to her when he had to study, or avoid answering the phone. Kathy continued to call him most every night, even during the six-week Bar Review he studied for to pass the New York State Bar. Elinor and Horace Hitchcock felt, as I did, that Peter could have made Law Review if Kathy had only left him alone.

Before moving, we were most happy over our decision to get a dog since the Avon Road three-story house was considerably large and isolated up on a hill. We found eight-week-old Trippy, a beautiful long-haired, brown and white Shetland Sheep Dog at a local pet store in the Village. Because he was young, we were sure he and Inky, the cat, would get along. In the process of cleaning out the house, as I promised Elinor before her death, I would be alone most of the time during the day while Peter worked in the City. I welcomed having a companion...hopefully, he'd become our watchdog!

The move to Bronxville went smoothly. As it turned out, Trippy and Inky got along famously. Anne had a daytime job, and Kathy and I made every effort to make sure that things went smoothly. Eventually she moved into the City.

No sooner had we unpacked when I noticed blood in Trippy's stool. I took him to a veterinarian in Scarsdale, New York, after seeing a doctor in Bronxville, to get a second opinion. Trippy had worms found only in chickens! We learned that the breeder owned a chicken farm in Iowa. Regardless of the fact that he was registered with the American Kennel Club and had papers, we never bought another dog from a puppy mill or a pet store again.

Edie and Alan also left the City moving to Long Island. Soon after, she gave birth to a beautiful, handsome little boy. She found a wonderful woman, Joanne, to take care of the child while she worked in accounting in the City. We saw very little of Edie and Alan.

As for us, Peter introduced me to the Bronxville society where I met wonderful friends of his. We ended up giving, or attending, parties most weekends including dinner-dances. It became a tradition the Saturday night before Christmas that the Peter Hitchcocks would give a party usually for 20-30 people. In our invitations I warned them I would be serving something unusual...such a venison, goose, rabbit, or duck – all I had never cooked before except duck! It became a fun challenge. I enjoyed using Elinor's beautiful silver, fine china, and crystal. I always hoped that she and Horace were looking down upon us smiling as they entertained frequently throughout their marriage. I had fun decorating the downstairs of the house with Christmas cards strung on red velveteen ribbons hanging on the door frames of each room; I intertwined branches of evergreens, holly and red bows on the stairway banisters; our live Christmas tree was set in the back of the large living room, adorned with colorful lights, glass bulbs, handcrafted ornaments, and tinsel. Lastly, I decorated the fireplace mantel with its tall brass candlesticks, with swags of evergreens, glass bulbs, pine cones, and red ribbons. Usually we invited close friends, and out of towners. Once one friend, whom Peter worked with at Allied, and his wife came from Toronto, Canada. Just as our party became a tradition so did the Robert Evans' New Year's Eve party in Bronxville, which offered good company, dinner and breakfast after the stroke of midnight.

Upon Elinor's death, the New Boston house was left to Anne and Peter. One weekend when Anne and her beau joined us, we took a stroll in our neighbor's meadows after dinner. There were several horses and a pony at the time. That night we retired early. Nelson and Anne were talking in the living room.

"Goodnight, my Love," I said to Peter giving him a hug. We kissed and snuggled. No sooner had we dozed off when we were interrupted by a loud crash. The screen to the window on my side of the bed fell to the ground outside. I looked over and screamed. Jinx, the white pony, had nudged the screen and put his soft, wet nose on my face. He then let out a loud whinny.

"Annie," I shouted. "We forgot to close the gate!" Peter howled with laughter, which in turn made me laugh. I tried to push Jinx back but he wouldn't budge!

"He just wants to say goodnight to you," Anne kidded. "Stay where you are. We'll take care of him." They went outside. Anne led the pony back to the meadow, while Nelson attached the screen to the window.

We had many funny experiences in New Boston. Eventually, we bought Anne out, electrified the house along with installing a phone land line, and built the road leading from Beech Plain to our house. We no longer had to drive across the meadows!

*****

On November 9, 1965, I remember well the Blackout that hit the Eastern seaboard. Never have I been so scared being alone in our new home in the pitch black. Peter called that evening saying the entire City had no electricity. "Neither do we!" I told him. He was with his dear friend, Bill Knox – no trains were running. They would have to spend the night. As for us, Trippy, Inky and I slept on the couch in the sunroom with the French doors closed to the living room and the rest of the house. I had made sure all doors to the outside were locked. My flashlight went out and I had no portable radio!

Needless to say, I was happy to see daylight the next morning. The sweet, but oblivious, cat and dog slept through the whole night! Peter, in the meantime, came home as soon as the trains were running. Nine months later, after the Blackout, there was a baby boom!

In 1966, Peter and I drove up to Hanover, New Hampshire, for Gaylord's graduation from Dartmouth College. There we met Anne and Nelson and had a perfectly wonderful time. Gaylord then lived with us in Bronxville for a short period.

We decided to buy the Avon road house from Anne, Gaylord, and Kathy, having it appraised and taking out a mortgage. When that was accomplished, Anne and Gaylord moved to Cambridge, Massachusetts, where Gaylord worked for the First National Bank of Boston for two years. Anne eventually moved to Concord, New Hampshire, working with the handicapped. Gaylord then entered the General Theological Seminary in New York City. In the meantime, Kathy was found dead in her apartment after a three-day period. Peter had to identify the body, which was extremely difficult. The neighbor had smelled a foul odor in her closet and called the superintendent who discovered the body and called Peter. We cleaned out the apartment, which had been ransacked, because it was on the first floor and the window had been left open. In her medicine cabinet were bottles of pills – uppers and downers. We never did find out the cause of death. She could have taken one too many pills by mistake or committed suicide. Either way, Peter and I were relieved as she was in a happier place.

Soon after I had a false pregnancy after I hadn't gotten my period for six weeks. Peter and I were heartbroken. In the 1960's we didn't have pregnancy kits! However, we went to several specialists and learned that neither of us could have children. Our love for each other helped us to get through this. One evening, upon learning the horrific news, we sat down on the couch in the living room and talked.

"That means I can't have a child," I sobbed. "If you look at our baby pictures we both look very much alike – how I wanted a little Peter!"

"Darling, this is not the end of the world. We can adopt. What do you think of that?" he asked with a smile staring into my teary blue eyes. "But not a boy…we'd have the draft and armed forces to contend with. Regardless, I wouldn't want you to raise a child on your own if I am called overseas."

"You're right," I answered. "Oh, I love you!" I gave him a long hug and wiped the tears away. "Mother used to volunteer at The Cradle in Chicago, Illinois. She once mentioned that The Agency in New York City was wonderful."

"Then we'll talk to The Agency," he reassured me. "But no more tears."

"No more tears," I said half-smiling. "But I'm still upset. I know this has saddened you, too. You're always putting me first, so caring and loving. I'm certainly the luckiest person in the world to be married to you. But are you sure?"

"Call The Agency tomorrow to make an appointment. I'll meet you there preferably in the late afternoon. Now let's make this unhappiness go away," he continued. He took me into his arms and kissed me on the lips.

"Oh, I don't know…not yet," I whispered and gazed into his sparkling eyes. "I love, love, love you…but!"

"Shhhhh!" he whispered back and kissed me. The chemistry between us was extraordinary. I couldn't help but melt into his arms. Soon we entered into the world of Inanity. The bad news of not being able to have children faded away for the moment.

*****

I followed through the next morning with The Adoption Agency. As agreed, Peter and I met several days later. One interview led to many, many interviews for a year. During this time our sponsor came out to Bronxville to see our home and where our baby would sleep. She was most impressed. We were excited. The Agency was wonderful to work with and they got to know us well.

On a Friday we received the wonderful news – our 7 lb. 5 oz., 19 inches tall, three-week-old baby girl was born on September 2, 1967. We could pick her up on Monday. My sister, Barbara, mother of four boys, drove up from Princeton on Saturday to help me buy a complete layette at Best & Company in Westchester...bottles, diapers and so forth. She taught me tricks about sterilizing bottles of formula.

That Monday morning, taking the day off from work, Peter drove me to The Agency in the City. When we arrived, we were told to wait in the reception room.

"Sweetheart, can you believe we're doing this?" I asked. I was nervous yet about to bubble over with excitement. "I hope this dress fits her."

"Our life certainly will be different from now on having a little one around," Peter answered as he walked back and forth." He stopped. "It's wonderful to see you happy, Sweet-Love. You're going to make a great Mom."

"And you'll make the best Dad anyone could ever have!" I reassured him.

"Mr. and Mrs. Hitchcock do you want to come with me?" our sponsor asked. We followed her into the small receiving room and waited. She soon returned holding a bundle in her arms – a baby wrapped in a white blanket with only her tiny face showing.

"You want to hold her?" she asked looking at me.

"Yes...yes," I beamed. "Peter look at her. She's adorable!" She had light brown hair, which I stroked giving her a kiss on her forehead. In return she cooed. "Sweetheart, she's absolutely beautiful. Here you hold her but watch her head." Peter beamed too, taking her into his arms. He had such a broad grin on his face which made me smile. I know he was happy.

"Yes, you're a beautiful baby girl...our little Sharon." She cooed again. "Yes, I think we're going to get along nicely. Thank you for all your help," he said proudly to the sponsor.

"Yes, thank you," I agreed. "I can't get over how perfect she is." While I changed her into the little white lace dress I had brought, she stared into my eyes. I couldn't believe it. She was a happy baby! The sponsor gave us several bottles of formula to get started and a short history of Sharon: Her mother did not want to give her up. She and the father were in college. They were too young to get married. She was of English decent and an Episcopalian…as we were, though I had a little Dutch in my background.

We left soon after returning to Bronxville. Our next door neighbor, who happened to be unpacking groceries from her car, came over to us at our garage. She knew we were adopting. "Ceci, she looks just like you! What a gorgeous baby," she said. We were now proud parents.

Never once did our darling Sharon Myers Hitchcock cry. I gave her a warmed bottle of formula and put her down for a nap. We had lunch and took a short nap ourselves. I knew I'd be up all night. It was an adjustment for both of us. But because I was now a stay-at-home Mom, I never asked Peter to change diapers, unless an emergency, or to help feed her in the future.

We were lucky! At first I had feedings in the middle of the night and at four in the morning. However, I found myself getting up frequently to check on her. I would sneak back into bed without waking Peter. Needless to say, I got little sleep. Gradually she began to sleep through the night. We three would get up at the same time in the mornings. While Peter got ready for work, I fed Sharon a bottle. I then would make him breakfast which he gobbled up quickly, kissed me, and raced down the steps to the street, waiting for "Sal," the bus driver, to pick him up. "Sal" made special stops for the regulars commuting into the City. It certainly was convenient.

*****

In April 1968, six months later and the Saturday before Easter, Sharon would be christened at the five pm service at Christ Church in Bronxville. Our minister, Father Ferris, came over for a short visit that afternoon. Peter and I greeted him at the front door and invited him into the living room. The three of us sat down.

"I'm sure you've heard the sad news about Martin Luther King being shot this past Thursday," Father Ferris sighed. "A dreadful loss…he was a great pastor and activist for our black people and America."

"Yes, a great loss," Peter agreed. "He worked hard succeeding with the Civil Rights Movement by addressing discrimination and fighting for voting rights and equality for all black people…certainly a turning point in American History."

"Such a shame!" Father Ferris said emphatically. We were interrupted. "Is that the baby I hear?"

"She is playing in her crib, after awakening from a nap…such a happy baby." I beamed proudly. My family will be arriving in an hour. We're having a christening party after the service. You're welcome to join us."

"That's very nice of you but I must pass. Well, you have lots to do," he said standing up. "I just wanted to say hello." You are the only baptism tonight.

You'll be sitting in the front pew along with the godparents. I'll ask you to come up and to repeat after me...follow your program. I look forward to seeing you."

"Thank you for coming," Peter said showing him to the front door. "Until tonight then." They both shook hands.

"Thanks again," I exclaimed as I started to go up the stairs to take care of Sharon.

An hour later Barbara, Sharon's godmother, and her husband, Bill, and their four boys, arrived with Grandmother Myers. Mother and Mike followed. Shortly after Bill Knox, Betty, and their darling daughter, Susan, arrived. Betty was Sharon's other godmother, Gaylord the godfather. Peter took care of the introductions, as I brought Sharon downstairs. Everyone thought she looked adorable in her long, white chiffon dress, yellow cotton jersey coat and bonnet, trimmed with a narrow band of white lace.

Soon after, we left the house for the service. Much to my surprise the Church was packed. I handed Sharon to Peter. He and the godparents went ahead of me and sat down in the front pew, while I greeted our friends, whom we had invited to the party.

Throughout the service Sharon played with our car keys. Needless to say, we were mighty proud of her. She never fussed, when I handed her over to Father Ferris, and while he put Holy Water on her forehead in the form of a cross. After the service, we received many compliments on how good she really was.

Our party turned out to be lots of fun. Grandmother Myers kept studying Sharon from head to toe, as Barbara fed her a bottle. "She certainly is a lovely child," she commented. Coming from Grandmother that was quite a compliment! Just as I finished unwrapping unexpected gifts, the doorbell rang...perfect timing I thought. It was the pizza I had ordered, which Peter put in the kitchen. We thought that would suffice as we had five children present. For the adults I served Quiche Lorraine, a tossed salad, cocktails and sparkling cider. For dessert, we had ice cream, followed by white cake, which was decorated with yellow roses and the inscription "Congratulations Sharon." The party was a great success.

*****

That Monday I received a phone call from our lawyer, Mrs. Schwartz, who specializes in adoptions. Peter and I were relieved to hear from her. The biological mother could have asked for Sharon back within a certain period of time. We, therefore, met Mrs. Schwartz in the City to sign papers the next day. At last Sharon was legally our child!

*****

One Saturday evening Edith and Alan invited us to their home in Long Island for dinner. There were two other couples whom we did not know. Joanne, the Nanny, was taking care of their son, now about two years old, I believe.

We got through half of the dinner, making small talk and enjoying each other's company, when Alan stormed from his chair and gave Peter a strange, harsh look.

"Are you having an affair with Edie?" he demanded. I put my hand on Peter's thigh, caressing it.

"No!" Peter exclaimed. "What's going on?" He squeezed my hand.

"Alan, she is not having an affair with my Husband…absolutely not," I said emphatically. I gazed over at Edie.

"It's O.K., Cecil," she said as she got up from the table and started to clear the plates. Not another word was said over this disturbing accusation, but it must have been embarrassing, I'm sure, for Alan.

The next morning I called Edith at work. "You'd better tell Alan, Edith, if there is someone else."

"There is, Cecil. I've fallen in love. I'll tell Alan," she promised.

"Good!" I said and hung up the phone.

Soon after, Peter heard from Alan. He apologized and said he and Edie were getting a divorce. We weren't surprised. Peter and I always wondered if she had been in love with Alan in the first place. She kept putting off the wedding.

On a happy note, both remarried. Edie and her Bob had a daughter. Alan was given custody of their son and met a wonderful girl. Alan once told us, "And I forgot what real love was all about until I met my beloved wife." They came to one of our parties. We had great fun. After the divorce, we saw little of Edie and Alan in the future; however, Edith and I kept in touch exchanging Christmas cards.

Peter and I had a hard time accepting their breakup as we had such fun with the two of them as a couple. How could this happen, I wondered. As for us, we were deeply in love, becoming soul mates. Our love was stronger than ever and the thought of cheating was inexplicable.

*****

The months seemed to fly by. We raised Shelties for a while. Lady Trudingham Hitchcock with Sir Tilden Trippingham had two litters. We only charged $50.00 per puppy to friends and to those we knew. We then had backyard breeding, much to our horrors…Father Trippy, and daughter, Troubles, bred. We immediately spayed and neutered but kept one of Trouble's puppies, that we called Tracer. We now had four Shelties and two cats. After Inky died, Barbara, my sister, gave us Buffer, a beautiful and friendly one-year-old gray cat, and Biffie, a black and white striped feline that we found through a saleslady at Lord and Taylor's in Westchester. We picked her up at the age of eight weeks in Lord and Taylor's parking lot! In the future Buffer lived to be 21, and Biffie 24. My secret was, as treats, lean chicken, turkey, and Velveeta cheese!

In 1970, Sharon was almost three when we adopted our second child from The Agency. Courtney Anne Hitchcock was five months old, a twin, and at first was an unhappy baby. We could do nothing to cheer her up. Our pediatrician put her on a low dose of Phenobarbital for a time. Whether it was because she was separated from her sister or she was allergic to milk products, we couldn't tell. She was put on soy. We tried to adopt her sister but she had medical issues and was unadoptable. As Courtney matured I had to teach her how to climb up in the crib, crawl, and walk. Finally, we bought a "Jolly Jumper" that was attached to the top of a door frame...she adored it which made Peter and me extremely relieved and happy!

At story time before bed, we would read a book about adoption. The girls knew from the beginning that they were adopted.

*****

Peter was a devoted and wonderful father. He spent as much time as possible giving Daddy-Daughter walks when the girls were little. He'd put one child on his shoulders and say goodnight to objects, such as a lamp, a hobbyhorse, a photograph of Uncle Gaylord, and so forth. This helped to increase vocabulary. Great fun was looking out the window and identifying possibly an airplane, a bird nesting in a tree, a boy riding a bike, or someone walking a dog, etc.

As the girls grew older, he was a caring father always making sure they were loved and special. Not because they were adopted, but because he adored them, as I did. He was encouraging, supportive, patient, and generous. As a family man, he always put us first by working hard and making sure we were provided for and happy. We had "glows and glums" with the girls but that was normal raising children.

The year 1972 was a busy year for the Hitchcocks. Gaylord was ordained to the Priesthood on January 5$^{th}$ at The Church of the Resurrection in New York City. In the future he would become Rector of Grace Church in Westwood, New Jersey. Peter and I were quite proud of him.

Sharon was now five, Courtney two. Dr. Stedman, my gynecologist, marveled at the way I accepted having a hysterectomy at 37 years old. It didn't bother me, or Peter, as we had two beautiful daughters. Devoted Aunt Anne took care of the girls while I was recovering. Two weeks later I was accepted into the Junior League of Bronxville, which I immediately had to rule out because of the sudden news that Allied Chemical was moving to Morristown, New Jersey...and I was recovering from invasive surgery!

Associates of Peter mentioned that Mountain Lakes was a beautiful town with an excellent school system; thus, we had to go the next weekend to scout the area and find a house. We found a unique community of homes hidden in the woods surrounded by six lakes...family oriented and a haven to raise children. We bought a ranch, which I still miss to this day, on Laurel Hill Road, a prime area, for $69,000.00 (now costing over a million)! Thank goodness Allied moved us. As for the Avon Road house, that sold in a day!

No sooner had we arrived in Mountain Lakes when I received an invitation to become Treasurer of the St. Peter's Episcopal Church Women; thus, began a new career for me. I eventually worked my way up from Treasurer, to Vice-President in charge of programming, to President for a short time in the eight years we were in Mountain Lakes. Peter did very little traveling, which was nice, but worked on Antitrust. He also enjoyed working around the house without being asked! He did, however, become interested in politics becoming President of the Republican Party of Mountain Lakes, which was quite active. I became involved with Noah's Ark Animal Shelter fostering dogs and cats. At one time we had seven cats, five dogs, four gerbils (Mary and Noel, and Snoopy and Woodstock), two guinea pigs (Prika and Pepper), a rabbit (Thumper), not to mention the monkey (Lucky). The latter was adopted from a medical laboratory where Anne was employed. He didn't last long in our household as he would grab our clothing or urinate on us as we passed his enormous cage...quite unpleasant! We found a boy, through a wonderful pet store, who wanted a monkey. We were told by the owner that he walked out of the store with Lucky on his shoulders.

I did all that a mother would do raising children...Brownies, Girl Scouts, Class Mother, shows in New York City, and so forth. Courtney once mentioned years later, "You never sat down, Mom."

Sharon did well in school, while we had trouble with Courtney. She loved preschool but was always being put on a chair for "time-out." At Wildwood Elementary School she became the class clown, disrupting the class, ending up frequently in the Principal's office. We received many a phone call. Finally, we were advised to have her tested, which we did, learning that she qualified for State aide three times a week. Peter and I were thankful as she needed this training badly. As a result, Courtney's grades were much higher and she was happier!

******

After dinner one evening, I received a phone call from Phillip Morehouse, much to my surprise!

"Lee, how are you?" he asked. "I called your mother to get your phone number."

"Allied Chemical moved to Morristown. We're here in Mountain Lakes, New Jersey," I replied. "We're fine. We have two daughters now. How are you doing?"

"I've been married for twelve years," he answered. "We have two girls: Deborah and Sharon."

"What a coincidence!" I laughed. "Our oldest daughter is named Sharon and our youngest Courtney, whom we almost named Deborah, after Peter's aunt."

"I guess great minds think alike!" he laughed. "We're moving to Seattle, Washington shortly, where I have been named CEO of a company.

"Congratulations, Phillip. You've earned it by working hard. I hope you enjoy your new position, much less Seattle," I said.

"Say hello to Peter," he said. "Come out to visit us one day."

"I don't know about that," I responded. "Goodbye, Phillip."

Just then Peter walked into the bedroom. "That was Phillip Morehouse. He took my advice, finally, and got married," I laughed. Been married for twelve years and has two daughters."

"It's about time," Peter said giving me a hug. "I hope he's as happy as we are!"

*****

The girls loved Mountain Lakes...swimming in the summer, ice skating in the winter, enjoying friends, birthday parties, singing in the choir, and participating in all activities a town could offer. We were a happy family.

Somehow, we managed to fit in weekend trips, a three hour drive to New Boston leaving on a Friday evening and returning late Sunday. Driving two cars, Peter and I would haul food, five dogs, four gerbils, and at one time "Thumper," the rabbit. Courtney rode with Daddy in the orange Vauxwagen, and I with Sharon in the ten-year-old red Ford Torino station wagon. We had many fun and exasperating experiences. To name a few: Climbing up the steep hill on Beech Plain Road in New Boston, the Torino's tailpipe dropped noisily pounding the asphalt road. It was hilarious. We solved the problem by using the five dog leashes, tying the pipe to the back of the luggage rack. Another time I had a flat tire on the Garden State Parkway in 95 degree heat. As I drove, it sounded as though a helicopter was flying directly above us. A State Trooper helped Peter unload everything from the back of the car to the side of the road in order to get to the spare tire!

Once we had "Thumper," the rabbit, out on the lawn one afternoon in a fenced-in area. That night we had scratching and howling coyotes at our front door. Then somehow "Woodstock" escaped from his cage. It took most of the day for tearful Sharon to encourage him to come out of his hiding place by putting food and "Snoopy" in the cage on the floor. We were afraid the gerbil would find a crack in the floor of the house to the outdoors.

Frequently, the neighbor's cows would break through the electric fence, cross the footbridge, over our trickling stream, and wander around the property until our neighbor herded them up our new road. We found them big and clumsy, knocking and pushing each other to get our attention. The girls loved to feed them bread.

Then one night there was a noise in the barn. Peter investigated finding "Clementine," the porcupine, gnawing the handle of the wheelbarrow. She had already munched on the garden hose. Peter wasn't too happy about this! For some reason, porcupines love human sweat or perspiration. Peter did chase the animal up the road before the dogs found her.

We took many walks too. We'd climb Snow Mountain to Uncle Ned's cabin, going up the Old Hawley Road, off of our road, to the old lumberyard and through the pines. Great fun was finding trails in the woods behind our house, marked by red and white blazes on trees, made by Anne and Peter when they were children years ago.

Once we found in the Thurston's goat shed Uncle Ned's other piano. G.G. (girl goat) loved to dance on the piano keys as proud parents L.G. (lady goat) and B.G. (boy goat) looked on! The girls had fun feeding them saplings from trees and bushes.

*****

In 1973, we enjoyed showing Sharon, age six, Bermuda, staying again at The Coral Beach Club, where we had a two-room suite. Courtney was being taken care of by our dear babysitter, Martha, who also was in charge of the animals. In Bermuda, The Aquarium and the Bird Sanctuary were a hit, especially the talking parrots and gorgeous pink flamingos. Sharon also loved sitting behind Daddy motor biking and getting dressed up for dinner. Weather permitting, we spent a great deal of time on the warm, pink sandy beach basking in the bright sun and swimming in the clear blue-green water, or playing with Sharon in the sand. It was a week's vacation Peter needed.

As the children were getting older (nine and twelve), I became a student at The Institute of Children's Literature in Redding Ridge, Connecticut. My instructor was Alvin Tresselt, an author of some 53 children's books. The only way I was able to take the course was through home study. Peter became my editor, which was fun. I was able to get published in the magazine, Young Ambassador. "The Big White Birds" was put in Braille, on tape, and in different languages. Peter was ever so proud of me and suggested I write a picture book, which I did…"Tommy's Goodnight."

*****

Sadly in 1976, Mike, my stepfather, was diagnosed with cancer of the throat. He smoked for years, a habit my mother tried to stop. They had just bought a lovely, three-bedroom, two-bath house on an acre of land in Pennington, New Jersey, and had a Leslie pool built. The Mercer Street house was much too big for them at this stage of life. I found myself driving down from Mountain Lakes to Princeton twice a week helping Mother pack and move. As Mike grew sicker, Mother hired caring and compassionate Anne during the day, while she became caregiver at night. The doctor, using radiation, missed the cancerous growth on his throat! Mother virtually got little sleep. I would take her out to lunch or to my sister, Barbara, in Lawrenceville, as long as I got home by three o'clock when the girls got out of school.

We all mourned Mike's death in 1979, at the age of 65. He was a wonderful stepfather and father, working two jobs, taking care of our family. His death was devastating to Mother.

*****

And then it happened! Our good life in Mountain Lakes would come to an end, and I had to put writing on hold.

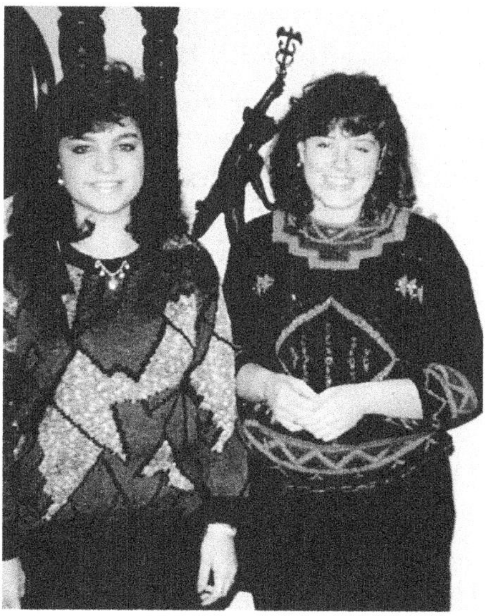

# Off to Houston, Texas

Each fall I would take advantage of the surplus of fresh vegetables which I would buy by the bushel at a farm in Boonton, not too far from our house. I would fill my deep freezer with blanched cauliflower, broccoli, corn, beans, and carrots.

One afternoon, around two o'clock, I was canning Jersey tomatoes when Peter walked into the house.

"Hi, Sweetheart, you're home early!" I exclaimed. "How's my Darling?" He never missed a day at work but would come home early if felt ill.

"I've been laid off!" he answered back angrily. "Twenty-one years I've given to Allied and…bingo…just like that, I'm let go." He clicked his fingers. I feel sorry for the other 1000 employees who were laid off also.

"So you weren't the only one…sounds like the company is up to something," I said. I stopped what I was doing with the tomatoes and gave him a hug. I stroked his wavy brown hair and kissed him on the lips. "We'll be fine…one day at a time. You'll find something."

"Gosh, I hope so! I knew I should have gone to Brian F's Company party, the new General Counsel," he remarked throwing up his arms. "Damn, damn!"

"But you weren't feeling well. We all had colds." I was trying to calm him down. "You didn't get laid off just because you weren't present at the party…no way! What is important is that we have each other. You'll figure it out. I'll be by your side every step of the way…even type for you." I laughed, trying to make him smile.

"Sweet-Love you're such a comfort." He gave me a hug. "Oh, I love you. I must admit the Company has been good to me by giving me one year's salary, an office and a secretary to help revise my resume, office supplies…everything to help me contact potential job opportunities."

"I have an idea. Let's take a walk," I suggested. "The girls will be home shortly. We'll be okay. You wait and see. You're a great attorney with a fabulous background during the twenty-one years with Allied Chemical. Could you leave a note for the girls while I put the jarred tomatoes in the refrigerator? Thanks."

Peter wrote:

> Sharon and Courtney:
> We've gone for a walk. Be back shortly.
> Love you,
> Mom and Dad

We climbed up Briarcliff Road, a steep hill, and walked around the long block making plans. Tomorrow Peter would move out of his office with my help. I would buy newspapers while he revised his resume. He would then contact headhunters whom his associates suggested.

The girls hugged us when we returned to the house. "Let's sit down," I suggested opening the freezer door and handing each girl a Popsicle.

Peter explained what had happened at Allied. "You'll have to help Mom more while she is helping me find a job."

"I'll help you," Sharon said. "Courtney will help too."

"Sharon you know I will," she scolded. "I'll help you, Mom, with the animals."

"Thank you," I said. "Now, how about homework?"

Thus, began a new journey for all of us!

*****

I gave up the idea of blanching vegetables for the winter and took a leave of absence from the Institute of Children's Literature. "Tommy's Goodnight" would have to wait.

While Peter worked hard trying to find a job, I typed letters to relatives and members of the Class of 1935, Mike's class. Perhaps they would know of an opening for an attorney with Peter's background. We followed up on ads in the newspapers but in return, received rejections stating that Peter, at 48, was too senior; thus, we were facing age discrimination!

The girls were wonderful throughout our ordeal. Courtney would always leave sweet notes on the kitchen table wishing us a good day, that she loved us, and had taken care of her gerbils. Because we were up late at night sending out resumes, we sometimes overslept. I'd lay out their clothes, cereal for breakfast, and lunch money for school.

The following is a precious note from Sharon I discovered years later which I have kept:

> "Dear Dad and Mom:
>
> I got up and all I did was cough and sneeze. I also have a bad stomach ache. I wanted to go to school but all I do is sneeze and cough and feel miserable. I hope YOU PEOPLE feel BETTER!!!! Lots of hugs and kisses. SHARON"
>
> (Sharon did go to school that day.)

Peter had many interviews. One, in particular, was with a company in Waterbury, Connecticut. He was being interviewed by a classmate of his at Princeton! We kept our fingers crossed as we would be closer to New Boston.

One afternoon Peter walked into the house deeply depressed after returning from his third trip of three hours, from Waterbury. "I didn't get the job. I was taken out to lunch, offered a martini, and was told I was too senior. What a waste of time!"

"Sweetheart, I'm sorry. Please don't get discouraged. Something will come up. You wait and see," I said trying to be encouraging, while trying to cover up my disappointment. "We have to go forward." I gave him a kiss on the lips and stared into his sad eyes. "I love you! As long as we have each other, we'll make it somehow."

Just then the phone rang. "Hello," I answered. "Is Peter Hitchcock in?" the voice asked. This is Margaret Whiteside."

"Yes, just a moment...Peter it's for you," I announced enthusiastically keeping my fingers crossed.

"Peter Hitchcock speaking...why hello Margaret! It's been a long time." He stood in silence listening intensely. Unexpectedly, he perked up smiling. "Can I get back to you? I'd like to talk to my wife...yes, I'll call you on Monday." He hung up the phone and said, "How about that! We're going to Houston, Texas!"

"We're what?" I shrieked from across the kitchen.

"That was Margaret Whiteside, the daughter of a friend of my father's. She's a headhunter...asked if I'd like to join an oil company in Houston? I'd have the title of attorney with no vacation for a year, but the pay will be more than what I was making at Allied. Sweet-Love, why not?" Peter asked. I was flabbergasted, stunned, and worried to say the least.

"Darling, moving to Texas? What about New Boston? It would be extremely hard on you...to start as an attorney...no vacation for a year," I said. "Money isn't everything! When do they want you to start?"

"December 1st...they'll move us...we can do it. Trust me," he said trying to be reassuring. He gave me a hug. "Let's treat it like an adventure. We'd be going out of our comfort zone by leaving our haven, Mountain Lakes. It will be all right. We'll adjust. We can even have a pool built!

"You're willing to do this for us?" I asked.

"Absolutely...it's a job! I'd be doing what I did at Allied."

Peter accepted the position. We had a month to make the move. Our Laurel Hill house was put on the market. Within days we were under contract for a February closing! We then flew to Houston to meet his associates and to find a house, taking our four cats in crates along with us and boarding them at "The Pet Bar," which we hated to do.

Luckily, we found a lovely large, white brick Spanish-style house. Returning to New Jersey, we rented a U-haul taking several pieces of furniture to New Boston and vice versa. I must admit I was quite apprehensive but tried to be upbeat especially with the girls...moving from a haven, as Mountain Lakes was, for city life? I had to trust Peter's judgment; thus, I began making arrangements and packing. The girls were excited that we would have a pool!

Mother drove up from Princeton in her blue convertible Ford Mustang, "Mrs. Puck," taking us out for Thanksgiving dinner and to celebrate our 20th anniversary at "The Three Sisters' Restaurant." We had such fun. The next night we stayed at a local motel, after having a delightful dinner across the street with our neighbors, the vonToernes. Their Renee would take care of the house until the February closing.

At the motel we were picked up early the next morning by a limousine that took us to The John F. Kennedy International Airport...all four of us...plus four gerbils in cages and four dogs in crates. It was a sight to behold!

*****

As the closing on the house on Pecan Creek Drive wasn't for three weeks, we had to stay in a motel which turned out to be crowded, chaotic but feasible. Because of traffic, Peter's short trip to the office turned out to be three hours each way! He learned to leave much earlier in the mornings and later in the evenings. He would come back exhausted from the trip alone but never complained. In the meantime, I registered the girls in their public schools and took them to our new house. I then became a chauffeur early in the mornings and afternoons. Sharon was most unhappy with the location of our house, which was in a subdivision behind an apartment complex, across the street from the railroad tracks.

Interestingly enough, Peter found out the company in Waterbury had been taken over, as was Allied, which became Allied Signal (now GE Honeywell).

At last we took title to the house. After three weeks in a crowded motel, we were happy to settle down in our new home. Soon after, we had an in-ground pool built with a diving board and steps, which we enjoyed on Christmas Day!

Peter began to work unusually hard. Sometimes he was called back to the office after dinner for a meeting. He also began to travel, with little notice. They were short trips, thank goodness, nothing like the trips to India! I got used to the frequent phone calls from the office when he had to leave – I would pack his suitcase, as he had to go that evening or early in the morning. As a result, I went back to writing a short love note each time, slipping it into his briefcase:

"My Darling:

I am so proud of you, such a brilliant and hardworking lawyer. I hope the company appreciates you as much as I do. Have a safe trip. Take care of my Darling and may God bring you safely back to me. Remember I am in your pocket. I love you,

Your Spoose"

I found myself being included in the many, many company functions, picnics, and social get-togethers. It took a while to get used to this lifestyle after living the quiet life in Mountain Lakes, New Jersey. I guess the change in climate played a part as our bodies weren't acclimated to the oppressive Texas heat and extreme humidity, much less, having to contend with the polluted smog. We had to put tennis balls in our pool's skimmers to collect the black soot!

I refused to donate our winter clothes, hoping each day we would return to the East, packing them in a cedar chest. I knew this was a pipe dream; thus, I began to treat our stay as an adventure, as Peter suggested, in our married life, bringing us even closer to one another.

With Peter working unusually hard, I became the disciplinarian for a time, which I did not like, as we had two rebellious children. Peter and I felt that going to the Episcopal Church of the Holy Spirit on Sundays would help. At first, we'd bribe the girls, so to speak, by taking them to our favorite "Steak and Ale" after each service. The restaurant had the most inviting salad bar and outstanding prime rib. Eventually, this became a tradition. Both girls enjoyed the Church, meeting new friends and were confirmed.

At first, Courtney entered the fifth grade, Sharon the eighth. The former did not qualify for Texas state aid. We were heartbroken. As a result, she did poorly in school and got into the wrong crowd of classmates. One girl talked her into running away. They were found walking on the railroad tracks in Katy, several miles from us. The child's mother called warning me that her daughter might try this again – walking the tracks to Austin. I immediately got in the car and found them. Courtney apologized crying, saying that she really didn't want to go. She was scared. I grounded her anyway.

As for Sharon, she hated eighth grade, but luckily met a sweet and fun girl, Lisa Morgan. To this day they are best friends; however, when she entered high school she got mixed up with the wrong crowd. Her friends then are not her friends now. She isn't in touch with anyone except Lisa.

I started to pick up my writing and began with "Tommy's Goodnight." I was asked to rewrite the picture book, putting it in a different time of day, which I did, and submitted it again to the publisher. While that was happening, I wrote two more books over a period of four months, and found myself working with three editors. I was asked to strengthen the plot in one, and submit future picture books to the other as they liked my writing. I had to slow down because of our busy, chaotic lifestyle. Finally, I found an agent to help me, but it would take months before I would hear back from her.

In the meantime, I took Sharon to St. Mary's School and Junior College in Raleigh, North Carolina, where I studied. She was accepted and loved the school; nevertheless, upon returning home from New Boston with Courtney that summer, I found her upstairs in the house with a friend. "I'm not going to St. Mary's," she said emphatically. I responded by telling her it was all right, but she was making a big mistake.

*****

I will never forget the night in 1983 when Alicia pounded the Texax coast, hitting Galveston, and headed straight for Houston – our first experience in a hurricane.

We were awakened in the middle of the night by a turbulence of whirring wind, clamorous thunder, violent lightning, and flooding rain. I slipped out of bed, followed by Peter, and ran to the back door leading out to the pool and backyard. "Look, Darling, it's a lake out there. You can barely see the pool," I commented. I was scared!

"Don't go out there, Sweet-Love. It's too dangerous," he begged. "There's nothing we can do until Alicia passes." I grabbed a pile of beach towels and lay them around the bottom of the back door. "I'm afraid the water will seep into the house." Just then the electricity went out. Out of the blue there was complete silence outside, except for the serenating of ribbiting tree frogs.

"What's happening, Daddy?" Courtney shouted as she ran down the stairway.

"The storm has passed," commented Sharon. "Yeah!"

"No...not yet. The hurricane's eye is over us. We'll be ok." Peter reassured us. "Stay away from the windows though." Just then, there was a roaring sound of a train. It was loud and startling.

"Look out!" I yelled. "It's a tornado. Head for the covered stairway. We should be safe there." Raging, whirling wind and pounding rain momentarily flattened the palm tree by the edge of the pool. "It must be Alicia's outer bands that are hitting us right now," Peter said comfortingly. "It should pass soon." As it turned out, the twister hit the apartment complex in front of our community. It was a good long time before electricity was restored. We learned that over

70,000,000 homes had power outages, along with parts of downtown Houston. There, windows blew out of many skyscrapers. The storm caused billions of dollars of damage by the 115 mile an hour winds. It was quite an experience, and luckily our family got through it safely.

*****

As Courtney entered high school, she became boy crazy to the extreme of sneaking out every night at one am, after hearing the phone ring once, which would wake us up, making it difficult to go back to sleep. I knew Peter needed the sleep desperately; thus, I went up to Courtney's room one day, while she was in school, which I did not like to do, and found her diary. She wrote about the nights together with the Love of her life. We immediately put an end to their ritual!

Courtney did not graduate with her class but did get her diploma after attending summer school. She broke up with Tim and was accepted at Blinn Junior College, in Brenham, Texas, but backed out at the last moment. Peter was extremely upset about this! Sharon, in the meantime, went on to The University of Texas – Austin, majoring in History, and rooming with her friend, Lisa Morgan. Both loved the school. Peter, too, became a fan of the college, especially enjoying the football games. Rather than wearing polo shirts with "P" for Princeton, he enjoyed ones with the "U.T." logo.

*****

One Saturday afternoon, we went to our favorite jeweler and bought matching gold wedding bands. Peter thought it was a wonderful idea, since we had been married almost twenty-five years. This surprised me. At our wedding, he did not want a double-ring ceremony."Absolutely not," he told me. "I have my Exeter ring." I didn't push the idea, but kidded, "You just don't want to be branded as married!" We laughed. "Not true," he said.

Returning home from the jeweler, we sat down in the living room. I sat on Peter's lap, admiring the ring on his hand. "It looks beautiful. Now everyone will know you are married," I teased.

"That's alright. I love my Sweetie-Spoose! I'm glad I married you," he beamed smiling, his hazel eyes sparkling.

"Ah, I like that! You're such a Sweetie-Man," I sighed. "I love my Darling." We hugged and kissed.

"How about renewing our vows one day?" he suggested.

"What a fabulous idea. I'm proud that you want to wear the ring," I said and stood up. "How would you like to go for a quick swim? I should start dinner soon."

"What are we having?" he asked. "If it's chicken, I'll fix Poule a la Hitchcock. Do we have brandy?"

"You're kidding, of course. You want to cook? I'm going to hold you to it, Sweet-Love...and yes, we have brandy," I beamed, smiling with laughing eyes. "Let's go for that swim now."

We confronted our minister that Sunday about renewing our vows. We were told that we would have to go on a weekend retreat. That really didn't appeal to us at the time, as too many things were happening in our daily lives. We just never gave it a thought again!

The following is a poem Sharon wrote honoring our twenty-fifth wedding anniversary:

"LOVE AND KISSES

Love and kisses
Mom and Dad
How I envy you
Staying together for so long.
You both are so in love,
Am I wrong?
You give each other joy and
happiness
In ways more than words
express.
You taught me the meaning
of love,
Caring for each other in
Good times and bad.
Here's cheers to twenty-five
great years!
By Sharon Myers Hitchcock"

*****

As for New Boston, I must say that Courtney was wonderful helping me for two months every summer. At first, we flew up with the dogs for several years, renting a car. I then started to drive, stopping off in Hilton Head, South Carolina, to see Mother. She had sold her house in Pennington, New Jersey, buying a lovely ranch in Sea Pines Plantation.

Eventually, Peter was able to join me for two weeks at a time. Even then, he received constant phone calls from the office. His vacations were not restful. He became discouraged and depressed. "They just won't leave me alone," he would remark.

I worried about depression, as he developed it when he hit forty. Thankfully, the depression was controlled with medication, but definitely inherited, as his father, two sisters, and his brother had struggled with it.

How I hated to put Peter on the plane and stay behind in New Boston. We would talk every night, but we hated the separation. Our amazing love for each other was that strong.

*****

One evening in the winter of 1990, Sharon called us from Austin announcing that Henry Haynes had proposed to her! Sharon met Henry at U.T. We were delighted, needless to say, as he was bright, ambitious, and charming. We knew he would make Sharon happy.

The wedding was held at The Episcopal Church of the Holy Spirit with Uncle Gaylord officiating. A small reception followed at The Hyatt Regency - West Houston, where family, close friends, and a few of Peter's business associates attended. We were relieved to get through that Saturday, as Sharon got cold feet before the ceremony and changed her mind. Henry convinced her that they should marry after being together for six years. Early Sunday morning, they flew to the Caribbean for their honeymoon and decided to live in Austin.

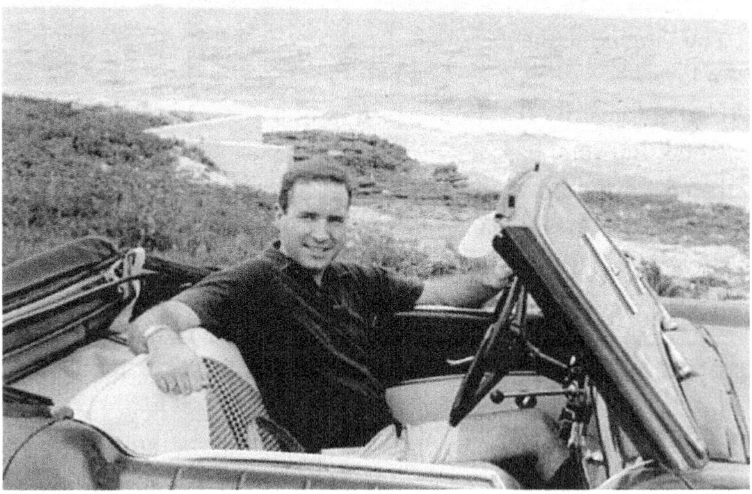

Peter in Galveston, TX 1990

# The Accident: The Trip to Heaven

Peter and I were faithful in having annual physicals and trying to eat right. That goes for eye exams, too. Both of us had to wear glasses – I for reading, and Peter for nearsightedness. Our ophthalmologist, Dr. Albert, who seemed nice, corrected our lenses several times and, of course, tested us for glaucoma, so he said. A concern of ours was the bright, blazing Texas sun. However, with some kind of neck issue, he was forced to sell his practice. It was taken over by wonderful Dr. Lee, who tested Peter for glaucoma during a routine examination and was horrified of his findings. A Visual Field confirmed that he had lost sight in a small area of his left eye; indeed, he had glaucoma and would be on eye drops for the rest of his life, and would eventually need laser surgery. We were furious! Dr. Albert left Houston in a hurry, so we found out from Dr. Lee.

Our bad luck continued on our 30th anniversary, on November 26, 1990, which fell on Thanksgiving. That morning I had had breakfast, walked into the bedroom, and went into vertigo with nystagmus. I could not walk. I had no balance. The room whirled around me, and I began to throw up. Luckily, Sharon was visiting and could help Peter. They took me to the hospital where I stayed for five days. As Antivert did not help me, the five neurologists were mystified! However, during my stay, I remember witnessing on television the space shuttle, Challenger, exploding in midair. That was terrifying and sad.

For a second opinion, I found another wonderful doctor – an Ears, Nose and Throat specialist. He diagnosed Benign Paroxysmal Positional Vertigo (BPPV), when I turned my head to the left, a condition, we think, resulted from a fall in Mountain Lakes, when I was filling a bird feeder and fell off a ladder, swinging my head to the left with great force. The doctor prescribed two milligrams of Diazepam to be taken at night. It evidently stops the vertigo waves in the base of the brain and cannot become addictive, if taken at that strength. He was right. I partially blamed this condition for my accident!

If that wasn't enough, one Saturday afternoon in 1991, I persuaded Peter to take a walk with our rescue dogs – Sharon's Chihuahua-mix "Chrissy," and "Penny," our puppy, a miniature Greyhound. Peter did not want to go. When I look back on it, I wish we hadn't. We walked down the main street of the community, Peter begging me to join him on his side of the road, which I didn't want to do. I gave in, crossed the street, just as a pickup truck whizzed by us. I moved out of the way and ended up slipping in mud, fracturing my right kneecap which almost literally split in half. During the six months, while the wired patella healed, the incision became infected; thus. I had emergency surgery, which weakened the kneecap. The Patellar Tendon atrophied, and I began to buckle. The same surgeon, a reputable doctor, who had two offices, was the high school sports surgeon, and practiced at three hospitals, changed the diagnosis the morning of surgery and removed the Patella, instead of repairing the Patellar Tendon, as promised. He never told me about buckling, how to use a cane, or fitted me with a brace. I learned the hard way! If I bent my knee while walking, I'd go right down, so fast I wasn't able to protect myself. This resulted in many falls.

Peter and I filed a lawsuit having the largest law firm in Houston behind me. They were aware of the doctor's reputation of malpractice. Shortly thereafter, I was dropped, when they learned that he was not insured during the surgeries! He was changing insurance companies.

Peter worked hard to find another lawyer, after I called several law firms – one was a famous lawyer, who was working on silicone breast implant cases. He wanted badly to help me, because he knew the doctor's reputation, but was too busy to take my case.

My new lawyer did a little detective work finding that my surgeon had five outstanding lawsuits. One was by a patient who broke her ankle. He had left floating chips of bone under the skin. We ended up, however, mediating but received little meaningful compensation; in fact, the doctor started at $1,200.00. We were appalled. As I write this book I have been in a brace for 24 years and will be for the rest of my life. But I can never thank Dr. Dozier enough for the hamstring operation (the fourth surgery), by putting my leg together, tying the upper part of the leg to the lower, as I ripped out all ligaments and muscles due to falls. At last, I was able to raise my leg up onto the bed, but not able to straighten it. What an impact this must have had on my family!

For months on end, I was on a bed using a knee machine or going to physical therapy three times a week. For the hamstring surgery, I had to sleep in a brace for five months on my back, allowing the leg to heal.

My darling, caring, compassionate Husband loved me as though nothing had happened. He was there for me every step of the way always cheerful and encouraging. He shopped, cooked meals, did the laundry, helped with sponge baths and even emptied the commode. On top of all this, of course, he had to work.

*****

Peter returned from the office one Friday evening to find me lying in bed crying. I had had enough. He sat down and held me in his arms. "What's this all about, Darling?" he whispered in my ear.

"I'm sorry Sweet-Love. I wish this accident hadn't happened to me. I'll be in a brace for the rest of my life," I sobbed. "I just don't want to live anymore."

"I don't know what I'd do if I lost you, my Sweet-Darling. Please don't talk that way," Peter said emphatically. Tears filled his eyes. "You're the best thing that's ever happened to me. I love you, Ceci." We both cried.

Wiping the tears from his eyes, he uttered, "Sweet-Darling, no more tears, do you hear?" He kissed me on the cheek, on the neck, and on the lips. The mystical chemistry between the two of us took over.

"Oh, what you do to me, Mr. Hitchcock," I whispered in his ear. He put his finger on my lips to hush me and wiped my tears away. "And what you do to me, Mrs. Hitchcock," he beamed with such a loving smile. "It's been awhile. Should we try?"

"Yes Please," I responded. Soon we again found Inanity – and for a moment I had forgotten my knee and the pain.

But he knew my whole life had changed. I couldn't jog, jump rope, or exercise on the bike. I no longer could wear heels. I had to wear long skirts to hide my brace, and I had to put my writing, again, on hold. I couldn't concentrate. I became depressed.

That night, while I was sleeping, I found myself being raised high up in the sky. Beyond, in the distance, was a light brighter than the sun and absolutely celestial. I then had to climb a hill. At the top the light glowed even brighter and was surrounded by a tall, gigantic wall. Behind this wall there seemed to be another world. I found a line of people, dressed in street clothes, waiting at a shimmering white arch-like entrance where someone stood draped in white. Behind him the lustrous golden light illuminated the background, where beautiful, peaceful music played. Could this be heaven I asked myself? I tried to pass the person at the entrance. He said to me, "You cannot come in. It is not your time. You must go back." Disappointed, I decided to walk down an embankment. I sat down on a large, white concrete slab with my legs hanging down. I was with another person, who was also turned away. Down below, I watched people driving cars on a tree-lined road, similar to the Saw Mill River Parkway in New York. I was looking down on Earth, I suppose. When I woke up I felt at peace.

Out of the corner of my eye I caught Peter, who was lying next to me in bed, admiring me in such a loving way. "You're beautiful! How's my Darling" he asked as he leaned over and kissed me on the lips. "I love you…you've been dreaming, haven't you?"

"Yes, and I love you more, Sweetheart," I said, kissing him back. "You'll never guess where I've been."

"I'll bite," he laughed as he stroked my blond uncombed hair.

"I visited Heaven!" I said smiling. I then told him about the dream – how it was not my time to be there. Those words have stayed with me, even to this day. They have helped me to accept the accident – to make the best of it – to be my cheerful self. I was thankful and lucky to be alive, and able to be next to my darling, loving Husband. I am sure it was God, who spoke to me, telling me to get on with my life. And I did!

Early Monday morning before leaving for work, Peter left a note on the kitchen table:

> "Darling:
> I didn't want to wake you up.
> Please take care.
> See you this evening.
> I love you.
> Me"

# Peter's Lawsuit

One Saturday in October, 1993, while I was driving the Chevrolet Malibu with Peter sitting next to me, I noticed he would flick two of his fingers on the left hand.

"Why do you move your fingers like that?" I asked reaching over and caressing his hand.

"I don't know Sweet-Love. I guess it's when I'm relaxed, like I am right now being with you!" he laughed. "Let's not worry. I'm just tired."

"I do worry…is it because of the office?" I asked. "You've been under such pressure."

"Yes…that is a concern. I have a feeling I'm gradually being forced out, probably because I'm sixty-two," he answered back. "Certain of my projects are now being assigned to other attorneys."

"Isn't that good, in a way, because of the pressure?" I asked.

"I guess you're right," he sighed. "But something is going on." I tried not to worry about the twitching of his fingers; however, in the past the girls frequently asked, "Why is Daddy so slow?" I pondered over this as I parked in our garage…and the office…that too was a concern. I looked at Peter. "Darling, try not to worry," I said. "Let's play it day by day." I tried to be upbeat, but I was worried just like he was. "I'm looking forward to having the Japanese Sushi we just bought! How about you?"

"I try not to bring work home…yes, let's go for a swim and then enjoy that sushi," he responded, sounding weary and discouraged.

"Good idea," I said enthusiastically, giving him a kiss on his cheek. "Ah…I love you!" He gave me a warm smile as he kissed me back.

"Me too!" he said getting out of the car. "You certainly know how to bolster me up."

Peter was right about the company! He was asked to quit, which he refused to do. The atmosphere in the office had changed leaving Peter unsettled and unhappy to say the least. He began to lose weight, wasn't eating, and had insomnia and hypertension to the point where he started to drink, because he felt unusually ill. Thankfully, that wasn't obvious and didn't last long. Our primary doctor admitted him into the hospital diagnosing a duodenal ulcer. After a week he was discharged, feeling and looking better, his ulcer healing. As a precaution, at my insistence, he attended several AA meetings but decided to stop. Because of the solid bond between us, he never touched a drink again.

One night after dinner, Peter was sitting in his favorite chair in the living room about to read the newspaper. "I'm proud of you, Sweetheart," I greeted him, as I sat down on the arm of his chair. "I'm glad we caught the ulcer. Alcohol doesn't take the pain away. It only makes things worse."

"You're right…I really don't miss it, anyway," he remarked. "I'm the luckiest person to have such a loving, sagacious, and supportive wife. I love you, Sweetie-Spoose!" He gave me a smile that made me feel ever so loved…" I remember the days in New York City when I worked for Allied, where martinis were served at our business luncheons," he continued. "A glass of ginger ale or a Coke was not acceptable. It was looked down upon…a sign of weakness. Here it is just the opposite."

"Yes, I remember, Sweetheart," I said giving him a kiss on his cheek. "And I love you, too. We have each other…remember that. We'll get through this. The company has no right treating you the way they have. You've worked too hard to let them get away with it."

"You're right," he said. "Age discrimination is what you call it. They'd have no problem replacing me with a younger boy, just out of law school for less pay!"

Soon after this discussion, Peter returned from work one night saying that the Company had asked him to retire which, of course, he refused because he wanted to work until he was sixty-five. It was now time to take action he told me…but how?

******

While this was happening, Sharon divorced Henry. We were saddened but, in a way, not surprised. On their special day she wanted to put off the wedding! After the divorce, she stayed in Austin rooming with a friend and got a job.

*****

Peter and I decided to change churches and began to attend a new Episcopal Church, recommended by Peter's brother, Gaylord, a Priest, who was a close friend of the Rector. We looked forward to Sundays, enjoying the services and making new friends.

One Sunday morning, during coffee hour, Peter met a parishioner, who was a partner in a law firm that dealt with cases involving Labor, ERISA, Employment and Litigation. Peter and Robert Wright became good friends. Thankfully, Robert said he'd be happy to take Peter's case, claiming Intentional Infliction of Emotional Distress and Age Discrimination.

Late one Friday afternoon, when the employees had left their offices for the weekend, I received a phone call from my Husband. "It's happened! I've been fired," he said, his voice trembling.

"I'll be right there, Darling," I assured him. "Don't worry. We have Robert on our side. Thanks goodness!"

I immediately drove to the office, parked in the garage, and entered the building – I'll never forget the silence. I could hear my own footsteps as I walked to the elevator. It was ominous, much less disturbing, as Peter had given sixteen years to the Company. But the thought of Robert Wright being behind Peter put my mind at ease.

"Hi, Sweetheart," I said, as I entered his office and embraced him with a hug. "They certainly want you out of here. They've even given you boxes and a dolly!"

"Hi, Love," he said laughing. "I'm about finished." I noticed that there was a person in an office down the hall watching our every move. Before long, we were loading the packed boxes onto the dolly, then into the parked Malibu station wagon and heading home. "Congratulations, Sweet-Love, you are officially retired after 37 years of employment!" I joked. We laughed. Peter would now call Robert as soon as we got home.

Thankfully, to avoid litigation, a settlement was agreed upon between the Company and Peter, claiming Intentional Infliction of Emotional Distress. Age Discrimination was dropped.

Not surprising, Peter found out that his position was filled the Monday after he left on that Friday by a lawyer just out of law school!

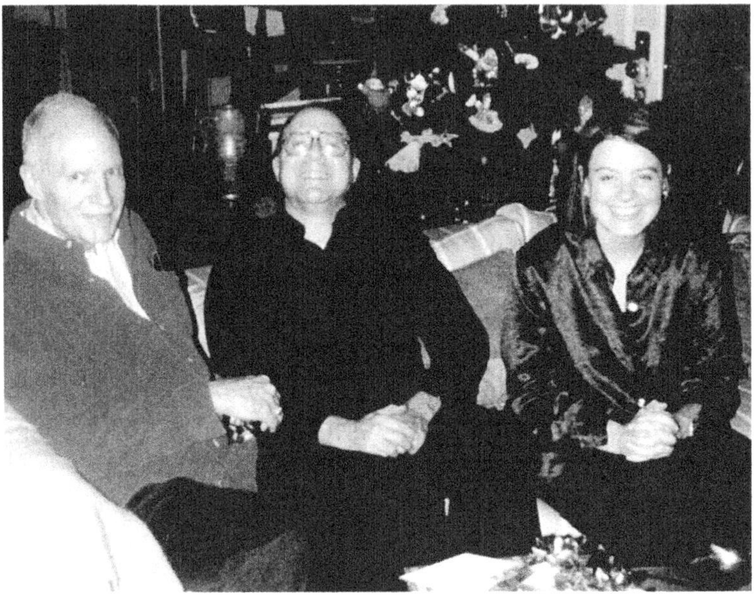

Peter with brother Father H. Gaylord Hitchcock and Sharon
in Hilton Head SC. 1997

# Part Five: Going Forward

## The Diagnosis

With unexpected saplings of "downs," Peter and I had enough of living in Houston. The girls were settled in their careers away from home, leaving us with the empty nest syndrome...we were now on our own and free to enjoy retirement. Deciding to downsize, we made the decision to move to Hilton Head, South Carolina, where Mother at 85 was living, a good reason to help her, if need be.

It took nine months to sell our house on Pecan Creek. During that time, we drove to South Carolina and purchased a Stable Gate Unit that backed up to the Equestrian Center in lovely Moss Creek Plantation, with its luscious and beautiful pecan grove...just before the bridge to the Island. We looked forward to walks on the Island's beaches with our constant companions, Penny and Meghan, in the wintertime...Peter called them our grandchildren. Like Penny, Meghan was a rescue, shelter dog. She had been left in an apartment by someone, or squatters, for a week with no food or water. Her howls were heard by a security guard who broke a window and took the ten-week-old frightened puppy, with virtually no hair on her back, to the SPCA where I found her. We had just lost Chrissy, our sweet Chihuahua-mix from bladder cancer. The veterinarian had tried chemotherapy and radiation to no avail.

Sadly, we lost both my sister Barbara's husband, Bill von Oehsen from Multiple Sclerosis, and Bill Knox, Peter's best friend from Bronxville, N.Y.

*****

On Valentine's Day, February 14, 1996, Peter presented me with a card which I have treasured to this day. It was printed by Carlton Cards for Ziggy & Friends, Inc. (1988):

"You'll always
have a place

in my heart…
… 'cause that's where
I keep my valuables!
Happy
Valentine's Day"
"To my Sweetiespoose, with
lots of love. May our love keep
growing, and our luck start leaping.
Me"

Bonded together as Peter and I were, our love grew even stronger moving to Hilton Head. We began to have fun, once again enjoying life. Mother, now remarried, was quite the entertainer, as she was in Princeton, New Jersey, introducing us to her friends…one in particular was our dear Frank Soule, who lived across the street from Mother, with his wife, Mary, who had Multiple Sclerosis. Frank and Peter became friends. Frank also became our financial advisor. We all went to many Yacht Club parties, enjoyed the Moss Creek Golf Club for gourmet meals and, of course, the Dog's Club, where Peter and I played Frisbee with Penny and soccer ball with Meghan out on the Point. There, members gathered for weddings, parties, or simply boated.

In 1997, a year after our move, Peter, now sixty-six, began to have balance problems. This worried me. After breakfast one morning in the kitchen, I kissed him on the cheek. "How about using a cane?" I asked. "I don't want you to fall, Sweetheart."

"No way," he replied emphatically, shaking his head. He began to laugh. "It's not that bad!"

"But your Grandfather, Dampada, used a cane. We have his collection in the china umbrella stand by the front door. Please, don't let pride get in your way," I begged. "You're being stubborn."

"Absolutely not!" he took me in his arms. "Will it make you happy if I go to our primary doctor?" he asked and kissed me on my lips.

"You know it would," I answered back. It's because I care and love you."

Peter did go to the family doctor, but was referred to a neurologist, whom we found to be kind, understanding, and compassionate. However, during the examination, Peter was asked to stand up from a chair, which he could do, and to walk across the office. I noticed he didn't swing his arms as he walked and took small steps. After testing him in other ways, the doctor announced that he had the early stage of Parkinson's Disease (PD.). "You have little expression on your face, a tightness. You're taking small steps when walking. I bet you have lost your sense of smell!" Peter nodded, "Yes." "It is believed that chemical toxins and metals in the environment could be a cause. They have an impact on brain cells which in turn lowers dopamine. The cells then degenerate triggering uncontrolled movements creating slowness, rigidity, and trembling. There is Sinemet, the drug of choice (Carbodopa/levodopa), which is converted into dopamine; however, you don't have the conventional tremors but you do have a bit of rigidity. I'd like to try you on Meripex for a while. It might cause nausea and make you tired but will help your balance. Always stand tall and bend forward as you walk…with PD. you fall backwards."

"Wow!" Peter sighed. "Who would think I have Parkinson's. Is that why I sometimes flick my two fingers in my left hand?"

"Yes, Peter, but Parkinson's isn't a death sentence. Rarely, do people die from the disease, usually from heart or other problems. You can live a normal and fruitful life, enjoying each day to the fullest. No one knows what tomorrow will bring. I want to see you in a month to see how you're doing on Meripex. By the way, coffee might help. It has a beneficial effect on dopamine."

We thanked the doctor and as we walked out to the tree lined street and to our new gray Honda station wagon, I put my arm around Peter's waist, my head on his shoulder. "That was a lot to digest, wasn't it?" I asked. "To think that Grandfather Myers had PD., in the 50's, but then died of a massive heart attack. It seems little progress has been made. Certainly more research needs to be done."

"Let's live in the present and not worry about the disease or what will happen in the future," he said trying to be upbeat. "Besides, we're spiritual. There is a reason for my having Parkinson's. Perhaps write about it. We're going to savor the time we have together no matter what, enjoying each day and each other."

"Wow! What a positive outlook…I'm proud of you, Sweet-Love," I said. Peter stopped walking and looked at me, staring into my cheerful blue eyes and said, "I love you." I gave him a kiss on his lips. "We will fight Parkinson's together…whatever it takes," I assured him smiling. I'll be with you every step of the way. We'll be fine."

How I remember the loving and wonderful talk we had in the car that afternoon: "We certainly have an amazing relationship, the way we bring comfort and joy to one another," Peter commented. "I am ever thankful to Edie and Alan for introducing us. It's almost as though we fell in love the first time we met. There was a spark between us . I wanted to kiss you outside St. Luke's Lobby door!" he laughed. "My tummy's now reaching out to you! You're my beautiful, sagacious Sweetie-Spoose. How about that, Mrs. Hitchcock!"

"And you know what! You're my Sweetie-Man…my handsome, preppy Husband, Mr. Hitchcock." We hugged. Peter started the car and said, "We'd better go to the pharmacy to fill the Meripex prescription. Just remember you're a loved Spoose!"

"Yes please," I said smiling. "You just wait until tonight." Peter's eyes lit up!

******

We loved our cozy Stable Gate, but after two years found it much too small and crowded with all the antique furniture we had brought with us from Houston. The dogs could not go out in the backyard because of the resident alligator, that watched our every move while rippling through the marsh, as did the water moccasins! We had to take them for walks on leashes; thus, we decided to move to a ranch on Saw Timber, offering us room for an invisible fence outside and more space to move around inside with its large living room, dining room, den, kitchen with a separate breakfast room, a screened porch that looked out to the golf course, and an office for Peter. We also had two bedrooms and baths and our wish come true, two-car garage.

Much to our horror, the day before moving, the urologist called Peter to say he had Prostate Cancer. He had gone for his yearly checkup several weeks earlier. His PSA was within normal range but kept going up and down. A biopsy verified the diagnosis. We were referred to an oncologist, but he'd have to wait because the moving van was due early the next day! Besides, Peter wanted to do research on the disease.

For a while, we settled in our new home. It was built by a couple who frequently entertained. The lady of the house developed Alzheimer's Disease and the husband several years later cancer. The house was sold to a couple who did a superb job of modernizing. The week before they were to move in, she had a heart attack and died. We began to have strange happenings, but that is another story.

We followed up with the oncologist after asking around and doing research. Peter decided on the Brachytherapy with Radioactive Seeds. We were told it had fewer side effects; therefore, he entered The Savannah Hospital for the procedure. By mistake the oncologist ordered half the dosage of seeds. We learned this at his office. "I made a mistake, but I am willing to give you 25 radiation treatments free of charge in return," he told us.

Little did we know about radiation and its side effects. After the twenty-fifth treatment, the oncologist commented, "You'll be impotent by the end of the year!" Needless to say, we were shocked as though we had been kicked in the gut. We were stunned, outraged, yet perplexed. In silence we walked to the parking lot and got into the Honda. I then reached over and gave him a kiss on the cheek with a hug. "At least we got the cancer...that's all that matters. We can still be close and cuddle," I said taking a deep breath. "And we have each other."

"That's true," Peter said smiling. "But we certainly seem to be having too many "downs" and less "ups." You're such a comfort, extremely understanding and encouraging. I absolutely adore you, Sweet-Love. You're certainly special. How I love you!"

"You're the same for me," I assured him. "Remember my knee accident and when I buckled, fracturing my ankle in New Boston? I could never have gotten through either of them without your help. My Darling, you too are a comfort and a joy. How I love you. We'll get through all this...we'll be ok."

We picked up Penny and Meghan at the house and took them out to The Point at Moss Creek to romp – anything to cheer us up! On the way back home we stopped at our favorite vendor on 278 and bought the sweet shrimp he had caught early that morning. Much to our surprise, he also offered the savory Bluffton oysters.

*****

Soon after Peter recovered from the Brachytherapy, we decided to help Courtney move to Bluffton from Houston, a small town down 278, the main highway from I-95 to Hilton Head. There we did most of our food shopping, attended a church on the Bay, and used doctors who had moved to Bluffton because of the traffic congestion on the Island.

Courtney met her future husband online. He moved from Iowa, and the two lived together before marriage. It was fun having them nearby, enjoying their company. Sharon too would spend the holidays with us, along with Peter's brother, Gaylord. Our family was frequently together again.

In the meantime, Mother and her Husband, Charlie, moved into a Life Care facility on the Island. She developed Congestive Heart Failure. Peter and I frequently would have brunch with them after church on Sundays along with Frank Soule, who had lost his wife, Mary, to Multiple Sclerosis. We all had fun together; however, Mother fell one Sunday as she left the dining room to pick up her walker. She had broken her hip and was rushed to Hilton Head Hospital – she also had suffered a stroke and went into the skilled nursing unit of the facility.

I found myself driving every day into Hilton Head to help her...32 miles each way fighting traffic! I developed Atrial Fibrillation, which was quite scary, and over time tried different medications to control it. I just needed rest and less stress. Mother passed away at eighty-six...luckily, Gaylord was visiting us for Christmas and was able to give her the last rites. Needless to say, Mother was miserable all the way to the end.

Also in 1997, Peter's youngest Sister, Anne, who was living in New Hampshire at the time, had had an asthmatic attack and was found dead by a friend in her apartment. Peter and Gaylord immediately drove up to New Hampshire to take care of the details. In the meantime, I developed tinnitus 24/7 and fluctuating hearing, had tests performed at The Savannah Hospital, and was diagnosed with Meniere's Disease!

That Spring Anne's ashes were buried in our New Boston plot in Massachusetts. She was extremely special to us, especially to the girls, Sharon and Courtney.

We stayed on in New Boston...Peter and I and our wonderful companions, Penny and Meghan. As usual, there was never a dull moment – something unexpected always happened. For instance, one afternoon on our routine walk up the road, Penny went ahead, Meghan walking beside us. Penny tried to chase a group of wild turkeys, all fifteen of them, in the tennis court meadow. The Tom stopped her dead in her tracks, flailed his wings, and chased her down the road where she joined us. We never realized until then that wild turkeys were extremely aggressive and protective of their young. Penny certainly learned a lesson!

Another time, thankfully, we left the dogs in the house as we wandered out to the Hitchcock meadow, named and owned by our neighbors. It was late that afternoon. The three horses weren't around. I commented to Peter, "They must be in their stalls in the barn." Out of the blue, we heard voices behind the line of pines in the distance, "Do you see them?" "No, Grandfather," a child responded. "Well, we must find them," the man answered. Peter and I were greeted by two adorable fawns. They allowed us to stroke the top of their tiny heads. The little buck with small knobs of antlers, pawed the grassy, weedy, wheat field, bobbing his head, and bolted into the woods, followed by his tiny sister. Probably they were being sought after by the grandfather and grandson who lived in a cabin not too far from us. We worried about the little fawns because of the coyotes, but never did find out what had happened to them. We were just happy that Penny and Meghan weren't with us.

And, we had our share of black bears, too. During the night one clawed the hood of our Honda, probably looking for food. Another poked his scarred head against the screen in our bedroom window awakening Peter and me. I slipped out from under the covers of our bed and cried "shoo" to the matted animal, to no avail. I then opened another window and slammed it closed. Bears do not like noise and are easily scared off. "That was pretty clever, Sweet-Love," Peter said laughing.

Peter and I enjoyed our "Thurtilperk Hill" with its fresh air, cool nights, and warm days. This year in 1998, October was exceptionally beautiful. We frequently took our dogs on day trips sightseeing around surrounding towns enjoying colorful fall foliage. We'd watch in awe as we drove through the brilliant Berkshire Mountains that were blanketed with seas of vivid reds, unique browns, golden yellows, and deep purples, the sun's rays glowing down upon the leaves making them even more dazzling.

We usually ended up at the Otis Poultry Farm in Otis, where we could by fresh eggs, maple sugar, freshly ground peanut butter, and their famous fruit pies, chicken and turkey pot pies, along with many other gourmet delicacies.

*****

Sadly, Dick Bauer, a classmate of Peter's at Columbia Law School called to say that Alan had died from a brain hemorrhage. We were unable to attend the funeral in Long Island as we were not given enough notice. We were in Massachusetts. This upset Peter.

*****

The beginning of November, as winter approached in New England, the nights dipped down into the twenties. Dinnertime brought many unwelcomed visitors...namely coyotes. Just the smell of food cooking would bring them to the house. Once a coydog, as the locals called it, arrived outside the kitchen door, while one stood at the footbridge, and still another waited out in our front meadow...all sending messages to each other through their eerie howls. I had forgotten to put the perimeter lights on around the outside of the house, which I asked Peter to immediately do. Thankfully, our dogs were with us, but that didn't keep them from being exceptional watchdogs. They would jump up putting their paws on the windowsills racing from room to room barking ferociously. All and all, we were able to chase them away, but we knew it was time to have the water pipes drained, and head back to Hilton Head.

# Unexpected Happenings

No sooner had we arrived in Hilton Head, when we received a letter from The Adoption Agency in New York City, asking if we would like to meet Courtney's sister, whom we tried to adopt but couldn't because of medical issues. The girls were almost thirty years old now. According to The Agency, it wasn't the biological mother's idea but Amy's. As it turned out, she stayed with Courtney and Rick for a week which became awkward and unsettling, according to Courtney who told us about Amy's unwelcomed visit! The two did not get along in spite of the fact that Courtney went out of her way to entertain her sister. Amy made passes at Rick, was caught going through his wallet, and wanted to sleep with Courtney after Rick had gone to work!

They came over to our house before they were to leave for the Savannah Airport. We all sat down at the breakfast table. Amy began showing us pictures of their biological mother who was married and had two children. Much to our surprise, Courtney looked just like her mother. From what we understood, she was battling colon cancer, which was good for Courtney to know medical-wise. Also, her grandfather was a dentist. Amy lived with the family for a while. She told us chilling stories of being bounced from one foster home to another. Once she was tied to a crib during a hurricane while the people in charge took off. She also talked about breaking up with an abusive boyfriend whom she had lived with for several years. They had a son.

We all went outside for picture taking. Amy then asked me, "Would you mind if Courtney leaves you and Mr. Hitchcock and comes with me?"

"Courtney can do anything she wants to. It's up to her," I said giving her a hug. "I'm glad we finally met you!" Courtney had no intention of going with Amy. In fact, the twins haven't kept in touch to this day.

*****

We believe the Saw Timber house is haunted! Peter and I tried to ignore "our Spirit" but things got out of hand. A neighbor told us that Nancy had died in the master bedroom…the original owner. That was not what I wanted to hear! I always felt as though someone was either following me from behind or watching me, especially in the night. Peter verified my feelings when he said he heard footsteps above him in the attic as he read or watched television in the den, usually in the evenings! Then after dinner one night while I was cleaning up the kitchen, Meghan bolted out of the breakfast room, with ears down and tail between her hind legs, and ran to Peter in the den.

"Darling, what in the world happened to Meghan? " I asked. The poor dog was shaking as Peter held her. I tried to calm her down by kissing and hugging her trembling body.

"Sweet-Love, she looks like she has been spooked," Peter remarked. "They say an animal can be scared by a spirit in a haunted house."

"Yes, I've heard that. It must be true!" I said. "Maybe it isn't Nancy, but the wife who was to move in but died of a heart attack. Don't forget the husband, who sold us the house, had placed a picture of her on the mantelpiece – could it be her?" The thought made me shiver. While we were chatting, Penny kept sniffing Meghan. "Let's all go outside for some fresh air."

"What a good idea!" Peter exclaimed emphatically. "I'll join you."

Not too long after this experience, I came down with the flu that lasted two months. Antibiotics did not work, including one for a viral infection. That made me extremely sick. At the hospital I was told that I had Viral Meningitis with a temperature of 105 degrees. Had I waited another day I would have died. I began to get confused and forgot what I was saying. After many spinal taps and a two-week stay, I was able to return home.

Soon after, Penny got an infection in her nose. The veterinarians couldn't figure out what was the cause, even though they did biopsies and other tests...much less wondered why she developed a heart murmur...no more frisbee for Penny...a condition she would have to live with for the rest of her life with the help of several medications for breathing! Then, Peter got ill with some kind of bug. Thankfully, antibiotics helped, but for a while, he was extremely ill, which worried me; however afterwards, one would never suspect he had Parkinson's Disease, as he was doing remarkably well with little symptoms.

We quietly celebrated the year 2000 at our home with Frank Soule, who was courageously battling bladder cancer. We lost our dear friend in early March. Realizing then that we had no reason to stay on in Hilton Head, we decided to move closer to Sharon, who was living in Princeton at the time; Gaylord, now Rector of St. Ignatius in New York City; and other family members.

We came across an advertisement in the newspaper, put out by Toll Brothers, about their building new homes in a 55-plus community in Jackson, which was located in the central part of New Jersey, and only forty minutes from Princeton. We thought about returning to Mountain Lakes but homes cost in the millions!

That spring we drove up to Jackson, staying at pet friendly The Red Roof Inn outside Princeton, which also gave us a chance to enjoy our family. We decided to buy an Extended Riviera Manor, consisting of two bedrooms and baths, a den/office, a kitchen with an island that led out to either the living room/dining room or to the breakfast room and sun porch. The 1,800 square foot house, with a two-car garage, was situated on less than an acre of land, on the corner of a cul-de-sac, and backing up to a state forest...just perfect for an invisible fence for the dogs. Mowing lawns, snow plowing driveways and streets, and shoveling pathways to our front doors were up to the Community's maintenance.

While our new home in Westlake in Jackson, New Jersey was being built, we had the Saw Timber house on the market, which was shown frequently but did not sell; thus, we moved in 2003, leaving it in the care of Courtney and Rick, rent free, until it sold. It was the worst decision we had ever made...a total disaster! "Our Spirit" must have spooked the two resident cats, causing them to urinate on the carpets and spraying the walls and curtains. On top of this, Courtney and Rick developed ring-shaped patches on their arms and legs...it was ringworm, which is caused by a fungi. They recovered in several weeks, but in the long run, did not take good care of the house!

We were eager to sell, of course, but in order to do that, we had to empty and paint the entire inside and replace the carpeting and curtains of the house. Courtney and Rick moved to Bluffton, while we drove down to Hilton Head, staying at The Red Roof Inn on the Island to supervise the cleanup! To this day, it is a sore subject with Courtney as it cost $8,000!

The house sold within two weeks...how happy we were to have a closing!

"Farewell...Spirit!" I beamed, giving Peter a hug. "I feel ever so relieved. I looked into his tired hazel eyes. "I love you, Sweetheart, and I can't wait to get back to Jackson."

"Me, too," Peter said grinning. "I love you, Sweet-Love. Hopefully, with a little luck now, things will turn around for us."

# Early Signs of Parkinson's Disease

Our move to Westlake was tiring, as most moves go, but for Peter it was especially trying. Meripex was slowing him down terribly. On the way up to New Jersey, we stayed at The Red Roof Inn with Penny and Meghan in Mt. Laurel, some twenty minutes from Jackson. Fresh snow had fallen that night, but we had no problem driving to our newly built Oak Hill home, where we met the moving van at ten am. The Community's maintenance had plowed the streets, including our driveway, and had shoveled a path to the front door. The movers came prepared, placing large pieces of cardboard on the oak flooring and carpeting within the house.

It was great fun watching Penny and Meghan playing in the snow, which they had never seen before. They'd jump, and they'd bump each other and fall into a hump…over and over again!

Luckily my stepbrother, Mike Morgan, and his wife, Babette, came over from Pennington to help us. While Peter and Mike hung pictures and emptied wardrobes of clothing, Babette and I unpacked boxes. As a "thank you" we all went to The Grille at the Westlake Golf and Country Club for a delicious lunch.

After the move, I worried about Peter as he was beginning to show signs of Parkinson 's disease. His balance wasn't good and he had little energy; therefore, we saw a new doctor, a neurologist, in Freehold, who took him off of Meripex and put him on a low dosage of Sinemet, which made him feel better. He did not have the conventional tremors but began to have more rigidity or stiffness, a type of Parkinson 's disease.

Peter never complained, was always optimistic, good-natured, witty, and a help around the house…always the Sweet-Darling I married! He never wanted to dwell on having PD., especially with our new neighbors. When asked how he felt? His answer was, "I'm coming along."

The year 2004 was hectic! We decided to give a catered, open-house with the theme of Christmas. I sent out invitations with a "P.S. What is your favorite cocktail? We aim to please!" Much to my surprise, everyone accepted…those in the cul-de-sac and in the surrounding neighborhood.

However, Mother Nature played a trick on us before sunrise on that day, blowing down a storm from the North by creating whining winds and swirling, stinging sleet, eventually turning into fourteen inches of snow. Maintenance neatened up the Community but plowed us in at the end of our driveway! This meant that our guests could not walk up to the house. Just as we were about to cancel the party, several neighbors came over and cleared the driveway, putting down "Ice Melt." Thankfully, the party was a great success, as were the special cocktails Peter prepared, the food, and hot cider served in large McIntosh apples...and as a result, it was great therapy for Peter! He liked our neighbors and felt comfortable being around them.

In March, I had a pacemaker implanted to control Atrial Fibrillation. It was a good decision because I do not need medication; however, I have had to become married to Coumadin, so to speak...a blood thinner that requires monthly testing!

That May, we headed up to New Boston to our "Thurtilperk Hill." Peter drove part of the way but started to feel uncomfortable and unsure of his ability to drive. He began to follow the white line between the two lanes of the divided highway until I corrected him. Then we drove over the Tappan Zee Bridge which was under construction.

"I'm not up to driving, Love," he said. "I guess it's the Sinemet. I get confused. I'm sorry!"

"You're doing fine. Pull over to the right of the tollbooth and park. I'll change places with you," I reassured him. "We're almost there...go slow and stay in the lane. Forget about the construction." For the first time I realized that Peter would never be able to drive a car again. This saddened me.

Peter pulled over and parked to the side of the tollbooth. We changed places. "I may have Parkinson's but I'm not going to let it get me, if I can help it!" he said unequivocally.

"That's right!" I exclaimed emphatically. "I sure do love you, my handsome, preppy Husband." He laughed which in turn made me laugh.

"You're such a comforting Sweetie-Spoose...I hope this isn't the end of my driving though," he sighed.

"For now anyway, Darling...for now," I said, trying to be reassuring. "Besides I'd rather be driving than cleaning house...anytime! There's a Rest Area in Danbury, Connecticut, but that's an hour away. We'll stop for lunch there. I'm sure the dogs will need to piddle."

"They're not the only ones," Peter commented chuckling. "Actually, I could use the Rest Area right now! It seems I need to go more often. I hope this isn't the beginning of incontinence."

"Not to worry...there's always diapers," I suggested comfortingly.

"NEVER...I'll use a urinal," he replied laconically.

"Well then...look down by your feet. It's in the red and white plastic bag," I said pointing to the floor of the car.

"How did you know I might need one?" he asked. "What a sagacious Spoose."

"At home I noticed that you visited "the little boy's room" frequently...go ahead and use it now...I won't look, but be careful!" I answered and laughed.

"Thank you, Sweet-Love," he said cheerily. "What a relief!"

*****

It was wonderful arriving in New Boston with its clean, refreshing air, and nature galore. We would be enjoying our seasonal home until the first snowfall.

I drove down our gravel road to the circular driveway and pulled up to the front door of the cottage and parked. The first to get out of the car, of course, were the impatient, excited dogs. Great fun was watching Penny and Meghan run free to explore the property, no longer confined by an invisible fence!

After we unpacked the car, Peter presented me with a card, created by "Shoebox Greetings," by Hallmark, that he had gotten in Freehold wishing me happy birthday. I was sixty-nine, Peter seventy-two.

> "I love you.
> I really, really do.
> Happy Birthday
> My Darling, this says
> it all. Happy Birthday to
> my wonderful Sweetiespoose.
> Me"

"What a surprise, Sweet-Love," I said giving him a warm hug. "You never forget!" That night we celebrated by going to the haunted, but renowned, New Boston Inn for dinner. It was originally built as a home in 1737 but became a tavern in 1760. Since it was Wednesday, the restaurant wasn't crowded, which gave us a chance to greet "the locals" in the Pub, who kidded us for being "Birders." We also were able to talk to the owner, whom we knew well, and who was famous for her gourmet meatloaf. We asked her how was "the resident ghost?" She laughed and commented, "She doesn't bother us but always plays tricks with strange happenings."

Years ago, as the story goes, a young bride, named Harriet, was waiting at the Ballroom upstairs in the Inn. She was dressed in black as was the wedding attire in 1805. A jealous suitor shot her dead. She has remained at the Inn ever since...is friendly and playful, especially with the guests. One can hear her footsteps as she walks up and down the hallways, fiddling with doors or she will remove a set of keys placing them in another part of the guest room. The owner told us that one couple spending the night was about to make love, when books flew off the bookcase. In 2005, another couple decided to get married in the Ballroom. During the ceremony the smoke detectors went off. The fire department was unable to turn them off.

Actually, while we were living in Hilton Head, we were thinking of buying The Inn, which at that time needed renovating and was run by two women. Our dear friend and financial advisor, Frank Soule, talked us out of it because of the cost. The Inn has had many owners: one was Florence Perkins, a well-known figure in New Boston and a friend of Peter's parents. To this day, the famous Inn is recognized for its beauty, architecture, history, and gourmet food. In spite of being haunted, celebrities Elizabeth Taylor, Richard Burton, and Bing Crosby frequented the place.

*****

We had to take Penny to our veterinarian in Great Barrington, about thirty miles from New Boston, for the infection she had contracted in the left side of her nose. No matter whom we took her to, no one had any answer as to how to cure the infection except to keep her lungs opened with medication. I literally had to take a tissue and pull the yellow discharge out. However, her spirits were high as she knew she was loved by Peter and me. She still chased chipmunks on the stone walls or up the apple and pine trees, and on hot days played and waded in the stream with Meghan. When we lived in Houston both dogs loved to swim in our pool.

*****

That summer, I had a wonderful experience. I had returned to the house from the post office and parked. I was wearing a red shirt at the time. I had gotten out of the car but had to retrieve my purse on the front seat. Just at that moment I felt something buzzing around my head. It was a Ruby-throated Hummingbird. It whizzed around the car and back to me again. I was able to greet the bird, which took its time to fly off. I still wonder to this day if this is the same hummingbird that returns each summer living in the lilac bushes outside our bedroom window. I had always wanted to hang a nectar feeder but was afraid of attracting bears! Luckily, we had many, many flowering plants and bushes that the Tildens and Hitchcocks had planted years ago on the property.

There is never a dull moment at "Thurtilperk Hill!" One afternoon Meghan happened to be sleeping in the shade outside the kitchen door. Out from behind the pump house, that bordered the woods, a large black bear casually lumbered over to her. She awakened in time to bark furiously. I ran to the kitchen, opening the screen door and blew a whistle, which I hung around my neck, hoping to scare the animal away. I then yelled, "Meghan come fast…fast…fast!"

The bear followed her, but I was able to close the windowed, kitchen door; however, the animal still tried to enter the house by pounding using his claws.

"That was close," Peter said holding his .22 rifle. I blew the whistle again. The animal just turned around and ran up the road.

"Wow!... thank goodness you didn't have to use the rifle, Sweetheart. It's not hunting season," I said, my heart pounding.

"I know...but it's ok if defending yourself!" he responded. "I wonder if that animal was a berry, grub or meat bear?"

"I think probably the latter," I said and laughed. I gave Peter a hug and kissed him on the lips. "I DON'T like bears!"

"Here...let's hug again, Sweet-Love. That feels good!" Peter sighed happily.

*****

Several days later Peter announced that he wanted to sleep in the guest room which was closer to the bathroom. I told him it was worth a try, if he really wanted to do this. He was becoming incontinent. As a result, the light in his room burned all night as he got up frequently.

I found myself very much alone after having him by my side for forty-six years...perhaps I felt rejected...certainly I was sad. I missed cuddling with him. Would my future be like this...alone and empty without my Darling. I tried not to think about it. "Go with the flow, Ceci, " I kept telling myself.

Peter wouldn't be in this situation if he used protection, but he was a proud man and would never ask for help, nor was he about to give into Parkinson's Disease! During the day, the Sinemet helped by giving him energy and confidence. He could walk without the fear of falling; thus, late one windy afternoon he decided to take the dogs for a walk up the road while I was preparing dinner. Little did I know, as he walked around the bend of the road, a tree came crashing down from the edge of the woods. Luckily, he jumped out of its path, thanks to his football training at Exeter, which taught him how to land on the ground without getting hurt. The dogs had been off having fun as he returned to the house. "It's certainly windy out there," he said casually as he joined me in the living room. "Sweet-Love, have you seen my glasses?"

"Weren't you wearing them on your walk?" I asked quite surprised. "We'll look for them tomorrow, Darling. Dinner is almost ready." I found a spare pair for him on the end table by the history books I had brought up from Jackson...I thought it was strange that he had forgotten he was wearing glasses. He needed to use them for distance.

The next morning we retrieved the glasses very near the fallen tree.

"Sweetheart," I said on the way back to the house. "Promise me that you won't take a walk alone, especially on windy days." I put my arm around his waist, my head on his shoulder. "I don't want to lose you!"

"Sweet-Love, I should have said something yesterday, but I didn't want you to worry," he commented.

"But I am worried that you had forgotten that you were wearing glasses while walking. You always wear them!" I answered.

"Love, I just forgot…from here on out we'll both take walks together…how about that?" he asked. Peter had such a broad smile on his face which in turn made me smile. "Do you know that you're beautiful?"

"You are changing the subject…but that's all right. I love you, my handsome, preppy Husband," I said and kissed him on the cheek.

*****

The first snowfall of the season fell the last week of October. Luckily, the snow was light and melted quickly. Having anticipated this, I made arrangements to have the pipes drained and the house cleaned…plus I had packed most of the car.

Peter began to have bouts of confusion. Forgetting about losing his glasses was just the beginning or "the tip of the iceberg!"

One morning I sat on the edge of our king-sized bed putting my jeans on, when the nylon quilt I was sitting on began to slip towards the floor taking me with it. I yelled to Peter, "Sweetheart, please give me a hand." He entered the room and just stood there. "Help me please," I repeated. "Give me your hand." He did nothing. "What is wrong with you?" There was no answer. He seemed to be in a trance. I knew then that he couldn't and frantically struggled by reaching for the blankets that were tucked under the mattress. I held on for dear life and was able to stop the fall, as I knew if I landed on the floor I could not get up.

I finished getting dressed and met Peter in the kitchen. I was shaking inside.

"I'm sorry, Love. I don't know what happened to me," he sighed. I gave him a hug and a kiss.

"It's ok…probably it's the Sinemet," I reassured him. "We're heading home Saturday. I think we'd better see Dr. McPherson, the neurologist, when we get back to Jackson.

"Good idea," he said. "I'll try to help you pack the car, Sweet-Love."

"That would be nice. I want to start taking care of your medications, just to make sure you're taking them on time, especially the Sinemet and eye drops for glaucoma. It is 30 degrees outside. Would you like a bowl of oatmeal and a cup of coffee?" I asked trying to change the subject.

"If you have evaporated milk," he said. "I'm glad you're all right, Love. That must have been scary."

"It was! Having the brace on helped," I answered as I looked in the cupboard. "We're in luck. There's one can left."

"Such a sagacious Spoose…you always take good care of me," he answered back, giving me a hug. "I hope my mind isn't playing tricks on me…I'll take a nap after breakfast. I don't sleep well."

*****

While Peter took that nap, with the dogs I drove quickly to the post office to have our mail forwarded to New Jersey. Steve was due at the house shortly. He was a young, talented carpenter with his own inventive and artistic business…a can-do-anything handyman and our caretaker.

I walked into the house only to hear Peter calling me. He was lying on the floor in the bedroom. "Sweet-Love, what happened?" I cried out. "Can you get up?"

I don't think so," he sighed. "I was heading to the bathroom when I tripped on my feet…I guess."

I was sick with worry. "Don't move." I heard Steve's knocking as he walked into the kitchen. "Am I glad to see you! Can you help me with Peter? He fell in the front bedroom."

"Hello there!" Steve greeted Peter. "Let me help you up." The tall and extremely strong man lifted Peter from behind with little effort, into a standing position. I thanked him and told Peter to rest on the bed for a few minutes. I was ever so relieved.

"It is a miracle that you came when you did," I commented as I showed Steve the small jobs that needed to be done, at his convenience, while we were in Jackson over the winter…an important one was to get rid of the hornet's nest outside above the front door one evening while the annoying wasps were dormant!

I said goodbye to Steve, thanking him again, and returned to Peter. "You should start sleeping in our bedroom using protection. You'll sleep through the night. I'll help you, Sweetheart. Seeing you on the floor was scary. Please…no more falls!"

"You win, Love…I'm sorry I'm stubborn," he said. It's embarrassing."

"Why? I'm the only one who knows the problem. You can wear boxers during the day. Besides, wouldn't you like to snuggle with Penny and Meghan? Peter laughed so hard he made me laugh. "Yeah!" I beamed. "Finally, you're listening."

# Accepting Help

Upon returning to Jackson, we immediately went to see the neurologist, Dr McPherson, in Freehold, who increased Peter's Sinemet to two times a day and put him on Aricept. "The latter will help his memory," we were told. The doctor also ordered physical therapy three times a week with an emphasis on gait training and balance. We faithfully carried out Dr. McPherson's orders for the next three months driving to Freehold, a twenty-minute ride from Jackson. There was such an improvement in Peter; however, his neck became rigid, meaning he was unable to turn his head to the left. Mike, the trainer and owner of the physical therapy practice, did wonders in eliminating the problem...so we thought as it would return.

Peter also had another problem which we had known for years. We had visited his cardiologist every six months to watch his Aortic Valve of the heart, which was gradually calcifying and closing up. I took him for an ultrasound, which led to an angiogram at Jersey Shore Medical Center in Neptune, New Jersey, a hospital known for its cardiology. It was discovered that the routine catheter they used barely went through the opening of the aortic valve; therefore, Peter immediately went into surgery to have a Tissue Aortic Valve Replacement along with double bypass surgery. It took four hours for the surgery, three of which the doctors had trouble stopping the bleeding! I was worried sick while sitting in the waiting room until the doctor came out to tell me he would be fine. What a relief! I was finally able to see my Darling an hour later. The anesthesia totally knocked him out and would affect him for several months. I was worried it would aggravate the Parkinson's. I was right! At first, he wore mittens on his hands so he wouldn't pull out the necessary tubes. Later, he was given a heart-shaped pillow which he would use to put against his chest for pain. After all, the doctors had to break the sternum in order to make the necessary repairs to the heart. On top of all of this, he was taken off the pacing machine which showed he had bradycardia, barely having a heartbeat. Peter was immediately taken back to surgery to have a pacemaker implanted.

I, in the meantime, went every day and spent several hours with him. Neptune was a good thirty minutes away. I knew deep down inside that he would have to be transferred to a rehabilitation facility. After a two-week stay in the hospital, he was taken by ambulance to Hawthorne Grove Rehabilitation and Nursing Home. Each day he got better with physical therapy...still his mind was affected by the anesthesia.

One afternoon, I met him in the hallway, accompanied by an aide. He was using a walker.

"Well, look at you, Darling," I said giving him a kiss on the cheek. Peter had a broad grin on his face. "You've certainly come a long way. I'm so proud of you!"

"Sweet-Love, I'm glad to see you," he responded. "But I want to go home."

"You will...I talked to the head nurse. She said you're doing exceptionally well but still have to learn how to use a walker. Besides, you'll get more rest here. You want to feel good when you get out, don't you?" I asked as we started to walk back to the room.

"Yes, of course," he replied. "I do need rest. I get tired easily."

"I'm sure you do. You've just gone through major surgery," I said as we entered his room. There was a chair outside the room by the door. "What is that for?"

"He won't stay in his room, even at night. He wants to wander," the aide answered.

Now I understand why the neurologist has taken him off of Aricept...because of confusion. I stared into Peter's sad hazel eyes. I was speechless. I never expected this to happen. I was worried about dementia, which goes along with Parkinson's. Trying not to think about this, I immediately helped Peter to his bed and told the aide I'd watch him.

"Love, I want to go home," he begged.

"You will, but you have to get rest. You can't wander around without a walker. You will fall. The nurse said you've been taken off of Paxil and put on Wellbutrin for depression. You should start feeling much better. Besides, your incision needs to heal." I handed him several history books he had picked out earlier at Barnes & Noble.

"Oh, thank you, Sweet-Love," he beamed. His eyes lit up. "It will give me something to do!"

"You'll be here for another week...then you can come home. Penny, Meghan, and I miss you. But while you're here an aide must help you. No wandering around in this room or out in the hall without a walker," I emphasized. "Do it for us. We'll be together soon."

I wanted to be with Peter more but physical therapy interfered. It was increased to two more hours every afternoon right after Peter's nap; therefore, I was only able to see him at four pm for an hour and then would have to take him in a wheelchair to the dining room where he'd join other male patients. I was not allowed to stay.

"Have a good night, Sweetheart," I said kissing him on the cheek. "I love you."

"See you tomorrow, Love," he answered back. "I'm one more day closer to going home!"

"That's right!" I said squeezing his shoulders. I'll see you tomorrow."

This schedule turned out to be very good for me. I was able to spend time with the dogs, do chores, and get more rest, which I desperately needed.

*****

Hawthorne did wonders for Peter. I brought him home a week later. He was a new person. His walking and gait improved as did his balance. Most importantly he had a positive outlook on life wanting to live each day to its fullest. He wasn't about to let Parkinson's get the best of him, especially because he got through the miserable heart surgery which he dreaded for many years. He was going to enjoy life with his Sweetie-Spoose!

I'll never forget what was said the next morning while we were in bed. I felt Peter's hand caressing my wavy blond hair. You're beautiful," he whispered. "I love you."

"I love you, too," I said half asleep. I looked into his sparkling hazel eyes. "You're my handsome, wonderful Husband, Mr. Hitchcock. I've missed having you by my side."

"Yes please, Mrs. Hitchcock," Peter sighed. "I wish we could enjoy Inanity. I'm sorry!"

"For what? Now, let's cuddle." I moved closer to him and put my arm on his waist, my hand on his chest. "Ah, that's better," I responded smiling. It was most wonderful being close to him once again.

"My precious Love," he sighed.

"Shhh!" I said. "Let's close our eyes and snuggle for a few minutes. I knew I should get up to give Peter his medications, but I wanted to enjoy this moment, as I knew it could be our last!

*****

I made a promise to myself that I would get more rest, as I was a ten hour girl, by taking a nap when Peter napped. That was my first priority. Secondly, I would let the house go if I had to, or possibly get someone in to clean, if we could afford it. I made up a schedule: I would get up at six am to give him his Levothyroxine for hypothyroidism; let the dogs out; help Peter to the bathroom; and climb back into bed until nine, at which time he would take his medications with breakfast. At night we would go to bed at nine, if possible. I was determined to make each day special. For instance, we took Meghan and Penny to the dog park most afternoons, usually after lunch and a nap. Peter would sit on the bench by the entrance as I walked the dogs around the perimeter of the park. It was fun to see Meghan and Penny bump each other, then jump, and fall into a hump until another dog intervened to play! Other days, we drove to Princeton or Pennington to visit with family members. Driving by 36 Mercer Street would bring back wonderful memories of our wedding, forty-five years ago, at Trinity Episcopal Church across the street. Peter and I wanted to treasure every minute we could to be together as we knew eventually we'd have a rough road ahead of us. Parkinson's was an unstoppable, progressive disease. We lived day by day bringing in as much sunshine as possible.

We enjoyed New Boston in the Berkshires that summer. I had help from a girl, named Carol Riiska, who was highly recommended through a friend of a friend. She would clean the house, eventually helping with Peter. His rigidity was worsening. He refused to go to the support group in Great Barrington, which offered physical therapy exercises in a pool. I finally had a script faxed from our neurologist to The Visiting Nurse Association for physical and occupational therapies, namely for walking, balance, dressing, and other exercises to stop the rigidity. At last, Peter realized he needed help!

After breakfast one morning I decided to open the front door to allow fresh air into the house. Much to my surprise, outside to the right, an acrobatic, friendly Black-capped Chickadee rested on a branch in the lilac bush. I greeted the tiny bird, calling out, "Hi...dee...dee...dee." The bird responded by repeating my call. I asked Peter to join me, which he did. The Chickadee swooped to the ground to a dandelion flower that had turned into a white, downy fuzz ball above its seeded pouch. If you pick up the fuzz ball and blow, its pieces will float every which way.

"Look on the ground," I whispered to Peter pointing. "The bird is picking up the pieces from the dead dandelion with its beak."

"I see...he knows what he is doing!" Peter said quietly chuckling. "He starts outside the fuzz ball and goes around and around until he hits the center never dropping a single piece with his beak...how clever!"

"He or she must be building a nest. The fuzz will certainly make a soft bed!" I commented. "I've seen birds carry small twigs to a nest, but always wondered how comfortable a stick bed would be for nestlings!"

"Now you know," Peter said putting his arm around my waist. "My nature loving Sweetie-Spoose...I love you."

"I love you, too, Sweetheart. Oh, do I ever!" I whispered hugging him. I kissed him on the lips. "Let's take a walk up the road. The dogs would love it."

"Good idea," he responded smiling. "A perfect day for a stroll."

We saw the Chickadee high up in the apple tree outside by the side of the house. "Dee...dee...dee," I called out as we started up the road.

"Dee...dee...dee," the friendly bird repeated after me. We laughed.

Returning from our walk, shortly thereafter, we drove to the post office to collect our mail. On our way, we found ourselves surrounded by at least twenty-five redheaded, brown turkey vultures. They soared above us dotting the sky, sat in trees, while others scavenged on the ground at the edge of the woods. We found out later that coyotes had killed two fawns. The birds flocked to eat off of the decaying carcasses, an eerie sighting I'll always remember in New Boston!

*****

We lost our sweet, adventuresome Penny in Jackson that November in 2005...our grandchild as Peter called her...a loss that was hard to accept. She depended on me as I nursed her for seven years with the nose infection she had contracted in Hilton Head. Her body just gave way at fifteen years old. We had her euthanized, for she had stopped eating, no matter what I offered her. Our hearts were broken, especially for Meghan. She howled in the car, as we came out of the animal hospital without Penny which in turn made me break down. We certainly will miss her. She was a great companion and watchdog. Interestingly enough, our new veterinarian in Jackson thought she had a fungus infection which was a shock to Peter and me. In our house in Hilton Head, Courtney and Rick had ringworm which is caused by fungi! Why other veterinarians couldn't have diagnosed this was a mystery to us.

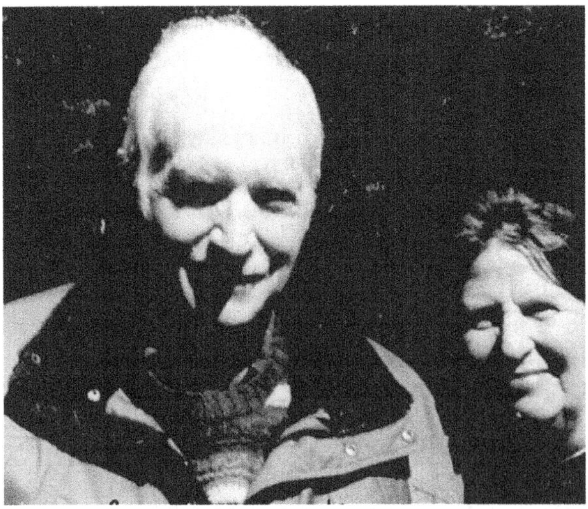

Ceci and Peter in New Boston, 2009

# Part Six: A Rocky Road Ahead

## Reminiscing

The year 2006 seemed to pass quickly. Peter was doing well with the help of Aricept. He was taking an interest in dealing with the mail, working with a new financial advisor, and making changes in our wills. At night, he enjoyed reading his history books.

After Penny's death, Meghan went into depression for about three weeks. She was subdued, not interested in food or toys, and slept a lot. Extra love brought her out of her shell; thus, we enjoyed her company while she savored the attention. A year later she developed cancer of the stomach which metastasized. We tried radiation, but chemotherapy literally took her life. That was January 2, 2007. To this day I miss the pair. They were wonderful companions, especially for Peter, who had a special way with the two.

We buried Penny and Meghan's ashes under the apple tree in New Boston, which was outside our bedroom window. Each had a plaque held in a metallic frame that glistened with the sun's rays.

*****

Much to our surprise, Courtney, our youngest daughter, found Lindsey, as we now call her, online at Border Collie Rescue, sponsored by Wag On Inn which rescues dogs and cats from kill-shelters up and down the Atlantic Coast. In Georgia, Lindsey was on the euthanasia table when she was rescued. Brought to New Jersey, she gave birth to seven puppies. All were adopted. We found the two-year-old extremely abused, having never been in a house before. Everything frightened her. She lay by the front door for a week…a leash was the only thing she knew; however, once she lost fear, she was docile, loving, and extremely bright, as we found out in New Boston that summer. There, we were worried she would take off but we realized she was totally bonded to us. To get her back to the house from her many outings though I'd have to honk the car horn and use my whistle. She was either taking dips in our stream, running down the hill or in the meadows and the woods, barking up storm…no animal would dare come to the Hitchcocks during the day!

In the meantime, Gaylord, Peter's brother, retired from St. Ignatius of Antioch in New York City. We were extremely proud of him. He took courses to become an Interim Minister. Eventually, he was temporarily assigned to a church in Hawaii.

*****

I would now like to introduce Jen or Jennifer. We adopted the ten-week-old puppy, again from Georgia and Wag On Inn. She's an adorable, long-haired terrier-shepherd-lab mix. Her mom was a small short-haired, black lab-mix as were her three bullying brothers. Peter called Jennifer a "pistol," as she was cunning, bright, full of personality, but domineering. To communicate she would growl – something we weren't used to. Our veterinarian said she had to have wolf in her. Perhaps so, but she was irresistible and absolutely adorable.

The dogs got along beautifully and were wonderful for Peter. He'd spend hours with them. When he wasn't feeling well, Jen returned love by lying on his bed next to him. They became inseparable. While Lindsey lived outdoors, Jen stayed with us in the house.

I learned through the puppy a little more about New Boston's wildlife!! Daddy longlegs, when aggravated, do indeed bite as will flying German roaches; pawing a Carpenter Ant is not a good idea for Jen was bitten on the leg...she loved to chase fireflies, mosquitoes, butterflies, dragonflies, and anything that moved in the air and, of course, crawled in the grass...bees on flowers, crickets, snakes, and toads...toads...toads!

Lindsey was relentless with porcupines. She tried to tackle four. The fifth she pulled down from a tree...for Jen one was enough! As a result, we spent many an evening in the emergency hospital in Pittsfield having quills taken out. We learned to put them on leads from three-thirty pm on, which is when porcupines climb down from their resting place – trees.

On one of Peter's good days we drove to Torrington, Connecticut, and traded in our 1997 Honda Odyssey for a 2007 model. Peter was quite the negotiator! As for me, I was delighted to have a new car with less than 126,000 miles since we traveled on busy interstate highways to and from New Boston. It was a good decision, for both of us were handicapped!

*****

I write from my Journal: "We're now married forty-seven years after a fantastic courtship of almost two years. I love my Husband. I wish we could go back to the way we were...no leg brace, pacemaker for me, and no Parkinson's for Peter. 'The Golden Years' stink! But we're lucky to be living where we are in Jackson - security, great neighbors and, of course, having New Boston – such work especially now with two new dogs. I pray I'll be able to do it all. I sometimes wonder, but I must keep going and take care of myself… rest… rest… rest; do your best; go with the flow and watch the stress I told myself over and over again."

As I mentioned, the dogs were wonderful therapy for Peter. He spent a great deal of time with them individually as he was losing interest in reading, dealing with the mail and so forth. He began to have painful sensations and tingling in his body. I again got help from The Visiting Nurse Association. They came three times a week for physical and occupational therapies, and to teach him how to use the wheelchair I used when I fractured my left ankle after buckling in 2000. The girls loved Peter. He was always cheerful by making them laugh. He never complained and was cooperative. It was amazing how he came out of his shell when around people!

Late one night I found Peter sitting in his favorite wicker, rocking chair in front of the fire I had built earlier. He was subdued and pensive. I sat on his lap, putting my arm around his shoulders.

"Sweetheart, a penny for your thoughts?" I asked giving him a kiss on his cheek.

"Sweet-Love, have you ever thought what it would be like if I didn't have Parkinson's?" he questioned with great sedateness.

"Or if I didn't buckle and have a knee brace! It's the same," I asserted…we're not 26 and 29! At our ages of 72 and 76, our bodies begin to break down," I said. "We begin to age. That's what I mean."

"Darling, we had a great time together, didn't we? I like to think about the days we were in school…oh, to be carefree once again," he sighed. We had such fun."

"We certainly did, but that was 47 years ago. We fell in love almost instantly, my sweet, handsome Husband. I have no regrets. Do you?" I asked giving him a strong hug.

"Of course not. I'm glad we're talking. I'm afraid I am a disappointment to you. To think that if I didn't have Parkinson's, we could travel, go to the theater, try different cuisines, and be with our friends," he answered. He seemed depressed.

"But we've done all that – we're slowing down and we still can have fun though and more importantly we have each other," I said trying to reassure him. "You can never be a burden. I love you too much, as you do me."

"I know, but it isn't the same anymore," he sighed. "I must say I'm glad we adopted Lindsey and Jenny…still I miss Penny and Meghan."

"I know, so do I, but we all can't live forever. Let's live in the present, always remembering the good times we had. Goodness knows what tomorrow will bring!" I exclaimed kissing him again on the cheek.

"But if something does happen, I'm not afraid, for I know we'll be together in the future," he said smiling with great confidence. I love you Sweet-Love."

"And I love you too, Sweetheart...we've had 47 beautiful years and we'll have more years ahead. Try to enjoy what every day brings. I'll be by your side and love you always. Just remember that. You're in good hands," I laughed. "I'll take care of you as you would me."

"You're such a loving, supportive, beautiful Sweetie-Spoose." He gave me a hug. "I know my life is becoming shorter now, but I just want you to know we'll always be together no matter what," he assured me. "We are Soul Mates. We're meant to be with each other."

As I stared into Peter's loving, hazel eyes, he kissed me on the lips. "Yes please...I like that," I said smiling. "But shouldn't we go to bed?"

"Oh let's not...I like making love to you," he whispered, stroking my wavy blond hair.

"Me too, my handsome, sexy Husband," I teased, kissing him back. Peter felt a spark. His eyes lit up! For a moment the world of Inanity existed but quickly faded away. I was aware of his disappointment and gave him a strong hug trying to comfort him. "It's getting late, Sweetheart. Besides, you have physical therapy tomorrow. Let's cuddle in bed."

"Shucks...back to the real world!" Peter scoffed.

*****

In bed, I wriggled myself over to Peter's side, putting my arm around his waist, my head against his shoulder. "I'm glad we talked," he commented. "I feel better...we should do it more often."

"We will," I agreed. "I love you, Darling. I'll dream about you if you will dream about me!"

"Yes please...I love you, Darling," he chuckled. "Good night puppies."

The house became silent except for a coyote's howl outside. Soon the four of us slipped into a peaceful, sound sleep.

# The Last Straw

As Peter's Parkinson's worsened, we made a big decision to move into an independent, assisted, and a skilled nursing continuing care facility. We wanted to stay together. No more moving! We, therefore, scouted the area, visiting various places, both in Massachusetts and around Jackson. We decided on Ashford Way, close to the Jersey shore. The wait could be one to two years!

Many of the facilities we visited were depressing: unhappy patients were planted around the nurses' stations; the smell of urine burned our nostrils which was inexcusable; and some places were overcrowded. At one assisted living, we met a patient sitting outside on a bench. He cried out, "Don't come here. It's not as great as you think it is – the care is lousy."

We got through the hard winter of 2008. I was definitely looking forward to returning to New Boston, especially because Peter began to sundown…a terrible part of Parkinson's disease. It would happen every afternoon around two o'clock where he couldn't sit still. He'd pace the floor, stare out the window, or simply fidget. I had never experienced anything like this before and learned to work with him with lots of patience! Sundowning can be caused by idleness, pain, boredom, or restlessness. I came across a plan that would be pleasing to both of us: I'd put on music…we'd end up dancing, which we enjoyed; I'd take him for a short walk before it got dark outside; or I'd put television on, especially "The History Channel," and serve a snack and a cup of coffee which has an effect on dopamine signaling in the brain; and I learned to serve dinner much earlier than seven pm, our normal dinner hour. All worked out! Of course, the food had to be easy to prepare but nutritional.

At last spring arrived, and we headed up to "Thurtilperk Hill." We would stay for five months. I knew the dogs would welcome the freedom to run without the canine fence, and I felt the fresh air and change of scenery would be good for us. Before we left Jackson, we went to a new neurologist, who put Peter on Namenda XR. His mind seemed to be clearer; he was more alert and interested in helping me with every day chores; and his mobility was better. I was always hopeful that the awesome man I married would come back to me, which for now he had. The doctor also increased his Sinemet to four times a day.

Thankfully, Steve had built a ramp from the driveway to the back kitchen door before we came up. This would help Peter with the walker.

We heard from friends that the population of black bears increased in the City of Pittsfield, an hour away from New Boston. The surplus was placed in the state forest on Snow Mountain that bordered our property. Great, we thought! Now we'd have to contend with an influx of black bears!

Needless to say, it was good to be back to our haven, "Thurtilperk Hill." Peter helped me unpack the car. I was extremely proud of him, for it was always an exhausting ordeal for me each year, as I had to bring up food to tide us over for a few days, along with summer and winter clothing for the five-month stay. Thankfully, we stopped off at a Burger King on the way up for an easy dinner…something we don't do very often.

That night, Jen now a little over a year and still "a pistol," as Peter called her, was keyed up from the trip. She wanted to play; thus, Peter was about to get into bed when she grabbed the sash on his pajama bottoms. I tried to stop her nonsense, but she continued to pull until his pants fell to the floor. We laughed until our eyes welled with tears. It was a sight to behold! I had to retrieve the pants from the living room.

No sooner had we settled in when our beautiful spring turned exceptionally warm. Happily there were no bear encounters! However, New Boston is grim and unpleasant during a power outage, especially at night! Not only is it gloomy and dark in the house but pitch black and shadowy outside with wandering wild animals! This time we had a lightning thunderstorm that literally lit up the house for a while. It was eerie! Luckily, we had lightning rods on our roof as we were at the end of the electric power line; otherwise, we would have had fireballs, which we once witnessed, dancing through the house!

Peter, unfortunately, developed a stomach virus which kept me up all night. The dogs were petrified, following my every step, while I helped him with the light from two flashlights.

As dawn arrived, Peter commented, "Gosh…I'm glad to see daylight. I'm sorry to have kept you up all night, Sweet-Love."

"You seem better, Sweetheart…thank goodness," I said yawning as I got out of bed. "I'm worried about losing food and will head into Winsted to buy ice. It's too early. Let's doze for a while." I leaned over his side of the bed and kissed him on the cheek. I then gave him his Levothyroxine for hypothyroidism with a glass of water.

"You know…I'm going to treat you like a princess when we get to Heaven," he remarked. "I love you, my Sweetie-Spoose." Needless to say, the words WHEN WE GET TO HEAVEN certainly surprised me!

"You're such a Sweetheart...and I'm going to treat you like a prince," I said smiling, as I put the water glass on the bedside table. "I love you, my handsome, preppy Husband. We'll be together always."

*****

Having had breakfast and giving Peter his medications, I headed to Winsted to Chris, the owner of the liquor store. He was kind to lend me a 5'x2' Igloo along with a smaller one, which he would rent out to parties. I had to buy ice, of course. Thank goodness, we lost virtually no food during the thirty-seven hours we were without electricity. Upon returning the Igloos, as a thank you, I gave Chris a box of chocolates.

We were wondering why we hadn't seen Patrick, the horse, out in the Hitchcock meadow. The cows were there but no Patrick. I know the dogs missed him. Later, we learned that he had wandered out in a snowstorm from the barn last winter and was found lying on the ground under his favorite oak tree. We were saddened, but happy he had been buried there.

In August, Peter began to take Coumadin, a blood thinner, because of his pacemaker and the possibility of blood clots forming...that turned out to be an enormous mistake!

One day we had finished lunch and I had cleared the dining room table. As I walked into the kitchen, I heard a loud, startling THUD! Peter had stood up from the table and keeled over, landing on the floor with the wheelchair on top of him. He was unconscious and bleeding on the left side of his forehead. I thought he was gone. He was unresponsive until he felt me gently patting him on the cheeks and hearing my voice screaming, "Peter...Peter." He opened his eyes and asked smiling, "Hi, Darling...what happened? Why am I on the floor?"

"You fell, hitting your head and became unconscious," I said. "Don't move!" I immediately grabbed a pillow from the living room couch and placed it under his head. I then proceeded to fill a bag full of ice, which I placed on his forehead. Luckily, the swelling went down quickly.

"I feel fine, Sweet-Love," he assured me and got up from the floor. I was amazed!

"Are you sure, Darling...boy, you had me scared. What in the world caused you to fall?" I asked wondering. "Rest on the couch for a while."

Soon after, we got into the car with Lindsey and Jen, and went to a produce stand on the way to Winsted for sweet corn. However, when we returned to the house, I suggested that he take a short nap while I prepared dinner. An hour later Peter awoke groggy and twitching his eyes and cheeks, not making sense while trying to talk. I immediately called 911, whereby an ambulance arrived taking him to the Trauma Center at the Pittsfield Hospital. There I remember being asked by the doctor over and over again, "Do you want us to save him?" "Absolutely," I told him. "Do everything you can to help him."

The diagnosis was a Subdural Hematoma on the right side of his head, the opposite side of where he was struck by the wheelchair. Thankfully, after many CAT scans and an overnight of observation, it was decided he didn't need surgery; however, he had lost the ability to talk and to walk. As for the hematoma, the body began to absorb the excess blood that was pressing against his brain. After several weeks, and physical therapy, he was transferred to a facility which was owned by The Hospital until there was a bed available at Birchwood in Great Barrington.

The trauma team at The Hospital felt he had suffered a stroke and possibly a seizure. I still feel, to this day, that he fainted from low blood pressure due to the increase in Sinemet; that the fall caused a stroke, as part of his right side of the mouth sagged; and that he was weak on the right side of his body.

All this time, I was commuting back and forth from New Boston to Pittsfield, and finally to Great Barrington. At Birchwood, with lots of love and encouragement from the staff, he was able to regain his speech and to walk with a walker. Still, he had to have more rehabilitation. Therefore, he was transferred to Ashford Way, outside of Jackson, while I closed up the New Boston home. We were glad he was accepted, as it would give us an idea of what the environment was like and how patients were being treated by the staff in the Assisted and Skilled Nursing Units. After all, we had decided to move to Ashford permanently in the future!

The care at the facility was all right; however, Peter hated every minute of his stay there. He kept telling me that he was going to find a way to escape, which I discouraged. He hated physical therapy and the hours he sat alone in his wheelchair, with an alarm ready to go off any minute if he tried to stand up. Seeing me made his day! I hated to find him at the nurses' station sleeping because of boredom. He had no one to talk to!

After a stay of two weeks at Ashford, he finally was able to return home. We were thrilled! In the car, Peter stated emphatically, "We're not moving to that place. You weren't there all the time!"

"I agree...I did find out from a resident that it is getting too expensive, as they were charging $10,000 a month for independent living," I said. "Let's not think about Ashford. You're doing well, but you must use your walker...no more falls. Please be careful! Do you promise?"

"I promise...cross my heart," he said and laughed. You know Parkinson's disease is relentless. My rigidity is getting worse and I get confused. But I know one thing...I love my Spoose."

"I love you, too," I answered, reaching out for his hand which I began to caress. "We'll fight Parkinson's together. As long as we have each other we'll be fine. I'll be with you every step of the way, as you would be for me!" He wore a broad smile on his face which in turn, made me smile. "And we won't be moving to Ashford Way!"

Upon returning to the house, I received a message on the Caller ID asking me to phone back Edith Bailey's daughter, which I did. I was told that Edie, who was a classmate of mine at St. Luke's School of Nursing, died of a massive heart attack in 2007. The daughter had a hard time finding our phone number until she received our forwarded, annual Christmas card. I had lost a dear friend. She and Alan, Peter's roommate at Columbia Law School, had introduced me to Peter.

# Home at Last

I had a ramp delivered for the front entrance of our house to be used by Peter with his walker or wheelchair, and a commode for the side of his bed, if he needed it. I found that Peter required far more care now. Luckily, he was able to stay by himself if I needed to leave the house…usually he would nap. We went back to the old routine of my getting up at six every morning, letting the dogs out, changing and giving Peter his thyroid medication which had to be taken on an empty stomach. I then would sleep next to my Love until eight o'clock, at which time, I'd give him Instant Breakfast in a glass of milk to take with his eleven medications to avoid nausea. He did not want any more to eat; therefore, we were able to sleep another hour until nine, at which time I'd fix breakfast and help him get dressed. Since Peter's retirement in 1994, we had a habit of sometimes sleeping until ten in the morning. Of course, in New Boston, that rarely happened because The Visiting Nurse Association would arrive at nine am most of the time. On those days we'd go to bed early at night.

On February 14, 2009, I surprised my Love with a special Valentine dinner offered by The Grille here at Westlake in Jackson. As Peter couldn't go to the restaurant, I brought the food to him. His eyes lit up when he opened the Styrofoam container which held surf and turf, a vegetable and a roll. On the side, we had salad, and for dessert chocolate cheesecake. Peter's reaction made me extremely happy as I wanted to bring in cheer as much as possible. Throughout dinner I had music playing. When we finished, we danced…a moment I'll never forget. I was surprised that he remembered the dancing steps but this was one of his good days. How wonderful it was being in his arms! Peter commented, "This reminds me of the night we danced the night away in Bermuda."

"Yes, at the Coral Beach Club," I said. "That was wonderful, just like now. I like being in your arms. I wish we could stay like this forever!"

"That would be nice," he sighed and smiled. "Thank you, Sweet-Love, for the Valentine surprise. You certainly are a sagacious Sweetie-Spoose." I gave Peter a kiss on his lips. "My sweet Darling, I love you so much," I said staring into his sparkling hazel eyes. Do you realize that 51 years ago we met for the first time in the lobby of St. Luke's? You were studying at Columbia Law School then."

"Yes...and you were beautiful, as you are now. I love you," he answered. "I wish I didn't have Parkinson's." I placed my finger on his lips to hush him…"Shhh!" I whispered. "Let's dance some more." I was extremely surprised that he remembered Bermuda and our meeting at St. Luke's. It was rewarding to me to see him relaxed and happy. It had been a good evening for him...and for me!

*****

Peter's sundowning got worse. As a result, I took him to our neurologist, who put him through a series of tests. She found that his brain "was slow;" consequently, she doubled the Namenda which helped enormously...still his dementia increased, which worried and saddened me.

And then I buckled! While letting the dog out one night, I tripped on the shoelace that had become untied on my slipper. My right knee buckled, and I landed on my left arm fracturing it. The pain was excruciating. Barbara Engler, a close friend across the way, came over to take care of Peter while I was being transported by ambulance to the Emergency Room in the hospital in Freehold – it was decided that I should go to The Rehabilitation Hospital in Tinton Falls for fear that I might fall at home, as I had no use of my left arm. How would I take care of Peter? Frantically, with my older daughter Sharon's help, we found a live-in from a highly recommended agency for $1,000.00 a week! With physical therapy twice a day and determination, I was able to leave the hospital in two weeks...still I needed help taking care of Peter. I used a local agency, which was unfortunate, as it hired young, inexperienced aides; one arrived inebriated after being with us for a few days. She had had a fight with a boyfriend; another girl, unmarried, having six children and living with "her man," stole money from my purse; still another used the excuse of watching the dogs outside while talking on the cell phone. We had had enough! We stopped the service as the fracture was healing nicely. It felt wonderful not having anyone in our house! With our determination, we got back to living as normal as possible. Besides, Peter was tired of tv dinners and waffles. We did learn a lesson though about agencies – do more research!

I would like to mention here that I will always be thankful to my stepbrother, Mike Morgan, who took me to all the doctors' appointments. Happily, after a week at home, I was able to drive a car.

Courtney, my youngest daughter, and her husband, Rick, drove up from Hilton Head leading us to believe that they were moving up to the Northeast where Rick would interview for a job while Courtney looked for an apartment. They had no intentions of moving and seemed to argue all the time. How lucky I felt about my relationship with my Husband. We had differences but always talked out our problems. Never did we wake up in the morning angry. We absolutely adored each other. Besides, I couldn't get mad at Peter, if I wanted to, for he was bravely facing Parkinson's with exuberance, dignity and grace, never complaining and always hoping that one day a cure would be found to stop the

Disease. As I write this, I am reminded that my Grandfather, William Starr Myers, had Parkinson's Disease in the 1950s...advancements have been made to relieve the symptoms but not to stop the Disease. We found that one must rely on Sinemet, which has horrible side effects. Peter experienced hallucinations, sleepiness, and fluctuating blood pressure, if he took too much. Sadly, Sinemet gradually wears off if you've been on it for a long period of time.

## The Turning Point

It had been a hard, nasty winter, snowing every other day in 2010. I did a lot of shoveling until my arm couldn't take anymore; therefore, I asked a handyman, I had hired before, to snow plow a path on the front patio and around the side of the house to the back patio…all for the dogs!

I quote from my journal: "In the snow, Lindsey would make snow angels. It was hysterical, but quite clever of her! She'd lie flat on her stomach in the deep snow, legs spread out – then she'd pull herself ahead with her front paws – roll her head in the snow right and left – with nose first, she'd continue to pull herself with her front paws, pushing with her back legs – she'd then roll over and flatten the snow. It was unbelievable! Jen picked up the idea, but not as precise as Lindsey – she'd then hop like a deer, attack Lindsey, lie down and stretch – then off she'd go running twenty miles an hour in between the bushes – back and forth until totally weary."

Sharon came for several weekends from Brooklyn, where she worked and lived, to help me find an assisted living community that Peter would be comfortable living in, if I no longer could take care of him. Just outside of Jackson, we discovered Beechwick that opened this past year. We did not do this behind Peter's back. In fact, he thought it was a good idea…just in case!

In March, Sharon was wonderful to take me to the Jersey Shore University Medical Center in Neptune for a new Medtronic pacemaker battery for Atrial Fibrillation. The original was six years old. How I hated to leave Peter and the two dogs. I worried that something might go wrong with the day surgery.

I do remember, on the operating table, almost passing out when the technician placed the magnets on my chest and back. That's how weak the battery had gotten! I don't remember anything more, but I do remember the Recovery Room where I stayed for an hour. The nurse was quite nice. I was then released, and we headed for home…what a relief. Of course, I was not able to put my arms above my head for two weeks and the incision was most uncomfortable!

From my journal: "Spring is here but for how long? At least in Jackson we wouldn't have minded because we have air conditioning but, here in New Boston, we use fans. On June 28, 2010, Mother Nature welcomed us with an extremely hot summer. Peter is not doing well – seems to be unsteady on his feet, has fallen – wants to sleep all morning, but having a hard time getting him to go to bed. Don't know if this will be his last summer up here – what about the future of 'Thurtilperk Hill?' It saddened me so much, I could have screamed. Have thought about going back to Jackson but Peter wants to stick it out…at least we have a breeze from being on the hill, and the nights are comfortable. Jenny tried to pick up "Mr. Toad," as I called him – she was sprayed and foamed at the mouth. It seems we have the same toad in the same place, by the kitchen door, every year. I warned her!"

"Lindsey attacked her sixth porcupine. The veterinarian pulled 36 to 40 quills. She was given antibiotics. We smelled a skunk this morning. It must have sprayed an animal out in the front meadow…the annoying smell stayed for several days. There's never a dull moment at 'Thurtilperk Hill'."

Early one morning upon arising, I began to notice that Peter's limbs were unusually stiff. He had a hard time moving his legs as he would sleep in one position, on his back, all night. To help, I bought a bedside railing which he happily used to pull himself up into a sitting and standing position. I found that sometimes I would have to put the wheelchair by the side of his bed. He could then sit in the chair.

I asked Steve to place brass handles on all door frames, in order for Peter to be able to grab one for balance if he felt like he would fall.

The Visiting Nurse Association helped me to understand rigidity. Peter had what is called "lead-pipe rigidity," a form of Parkinson's. His body would freeze like a lead-pipe, and his brain could not communicate with the muscles of his body due to lack of dopamine. The Sinemet had to kick in, in order for him to be able to move!

After a nap one afternoon, he grabbed the bedroom door frame handle. I turned my back for no longer than eight seconds to get a diaper, as I was about to change him, when he let go, falling backwards, landing on the floor. This time he couldn't get up. Rather than call an ambulance, I decided to dial our friend down the hill, William O'Brien. He and his grandson came up and lifted Peter, placing him in the wheelchair. His rigidity scared me. Other times, I would ask him to sit down on the commode by the bed. Sometimes he would fall backwards onto the bed. As a result, I asked my friend, Carol Riiska, who was a certified aide, to help me. She would come every morning giving Peter a sponge bath and helping him get dressed while I fixed breakfast. Later, she'd take him for walks up the road using the walker. I'd follow with the wheelchair.

There were times when I hated to see Carol leave for the evening, as I'd be left alone taking care of Peter.

Late one afternoon, we had a good but sad conversation in the living room. Peter was sitting in the wheelchair, while I sat on the couch.

"Sweet-Love, I'm getting too old for New Boston," he stated emphatically. "I don't want to come here anymore. This place isn't meant for a handicapped person. Can we go home?" I got up from the couch and gave him a strong hug and a kiss on the cheek. I broke into tears.

"I hate to hear you say this! What about the future of this house?" I asked wiping tears from my face. "I don't want to come up here by myself. Even if I could, you can't be left alone anymore in Jackson."

"Maybe we can go into assisted living," he responded. "Sweet-Love, I'm so afraid of falling. Parkinson's is slowly taking over my body. You need help to handle me...right...and I'm getting confused."

"Yes, Sweetheart, but you mustn't give up." Tears ran down my face. I hugged him again sobbing. "I love you," I whispered in his ear, "Please keep trying."

"Why are you crying...stop that," he scolded. "We'll always be together, just you and me...remember that. I love you...now no more tears."

"No more tears...I'm sorry," I said blowing my nose on a tissue. "It's because I don't want to be separated from you...I love you, Sweetheart," I responded wiping the tears away.

"I guess we should put the house on the market," he piped out clearly."Financially it's getting expensive to keep up. Besides I don't want you here by yourself!"

"I'm not sure about selling," I sighed. "I'm tired...let's go to bed and cuddle."

*****

We were able to keep our appointment with a neurologist, who specialized in Parkinson's disease in Pittsfield. It seemed like we were there the whole afternoon; however, we found the doctor outstanding and caring. He gave us a prescription for an Exelon ER patch. I thanked the doctor and drove to the nearest pharmacy in Pittsfield.

By the time we got back to New Boston we were exhausted. I was thankful that I had given Peter his dosage of Sinemet before we left the doctor's office for it had now kicked in. We had dinner, and I was able to put Peter to bed without any problems.

The next morning, when I put the Exelon Patch on his back, Peter began to feel strange and started to mumble, as if he was trying to get a word out. I called the doctor, who doubled the dosage. With that, Peter completely lost his speech and the ability to walk.

I called 911. An ambulance arrived soon after, taking him back to the hospital in Pittsfield. There they took off the patches stating he was never to use the medicine again. "Great!" I thought. "Peter's been a guinea pig!" He was again transferred to Birchwood in Great Barrington for physical, occupational and speech therapies. While this was happening, I began to quickly close down "Thurtilperk Hill" with Carol Riiska's help. How I hated to leave, but I knew then that Peter would never be able to return, much less come home.

He was transferred, by ambulance, to a skilled nursing facility in Jackson, where he'd stay for a month, as Beechwick would not have a bed until then.

How Peter hated the place! I agreed wholeheartedly, reassuring him that Beechwick was far nicer and very different. He would have to trust me. Each day I visited him; however, I would find him fast asleep in his wheelchair by the nurses' station. Other patients were moaning or simply staring at the surroundings. It wasn't a stimulating atmosphere. For lunch I'd take him into a small, crowded room where he was given food on a tray. Sometimes we waited for over an hour to be served. It infuriated me. Also, there was no place to walk him in his wheelchair except to his room. How we hated the place. What a beginning...if only I could take care of him...bring my Darling home...if only, I thought over and over again. How absolutely sad and defeated I felt.

Finally, I received the good news that Peter could move into the Beechwick Assisted Living in a week. During that time I used our handyman to move several bureaus, a television, an entertainment center, favorite pictures, and clothes before he was to arrive. When we got there, we walked into a lovely suite, which had two spacious bedrooms that looked out to a garden, a bathroom with a shower, a kitchen with cabinets, and a refrigerator. There was room for a table and four chairs which Sharon donated. I gave the Head Nurse a list of medications, along with a week's supply of Instant Breakfast to coat Peter's stomach. By now, he was taking ten medications: Acetaminophen for pain, Keppra for seizures, Lexapro for depression, Aricept for memory, Prilosec for an upset stomach, Oxybutynin for incontinence, Simvastatin for cholesterol, Zocor for blood pressure, Sinemet for Parkinson's Disease, and Levothyroxine for hypothyroidism. No wonder he was nauseated in the morning! And we'd have to wait sixty days for Long Term Care to kick in!

Peter was transferred by cabulance to Beechwick. I took him on a sightseeing excursion around the facility in his wheelchair, and then up to the Memory Care Unit which was for those who needed extra assistances, had dementia, or Alzheimer's disease. "Great!" I thought. They've put Peter in with Alzheimer's and dementia patients. I didn't say anything to Peter but I was upset; however, we were met by his certified CNA, named Bonnie, who immediately helped him get settled in the room. She then took him for coffee and a snack, introducing him to everyone. The girls were wonderful, cheerful, and caring. I was impressed, but ever so saddened that our life together was ending this way. It was a turning point in our marriage. Peter would never return home. We would be separated. I felt an emptiness...perhaps guilt, because I was abandoning him. It took a while to convince myself that I no longer could take care of him. He was much too heavy to handle, much less I needed a second person to help me. The house seemed empty not having him around. Thankfully, I had Lindsey and Jen, but I certainly wished we had Home Care, a very big mistake!

I made a promise to myself that every day would be special for Peter bringing in sunshine as much as possible. And I kept that promise. I began to see him around eleven am, have lunch with him, and spend the afternoon until three or four pm. It was a long day but I was determined to have a happy Husband.

Peter and I always expressed our deep love for each other by using pet names and phrases in facing uncertainties and challenging situations...because of his dementia I would repeat many things he would say in our conversations to buck him up...to reassure him in spite of our being separated.

I arranged to help with the physical, occupational, and speech therapists, which was good for me; as a result, I learned how to handle Peter. I would take him for walks using the walker, while I followed him with the wheelchair. Most importantly, we would talk on the phone at night.

Still Peter hated Beechwick. He'd sometimes get angry, which was not like Peter. He just wanted to go home. I began to use validation. I forgot about myself but entered into his world. Peter asked me one day, "What is the code in getting out of here, Sweet-Love? I won't tell anyone. I have to get out of here." I took him to the garden out back for fresh air.

"Sweetheart, why do you want to go home?" I asked comfortingly. "The girls are all nice. You're special to them. Don't you like them?"

"You're right," he answered back. "You'll be back tomorrow..same time...same station?"

"Absolutely...same time...same station," I replied giving him a loving hug and a kiss on the cheek. "Remember one thing...you're going to get better...but you have to be able to walk...then I can bring you home." I wheeled him into the dining room for the afternoon snack. "I love my Darling. We'll talk tonight," I reassured him. "I love you, Peter."

"Don't leave me...please...stay," he begged.

"Sweet-Love, I have to take care of Lindsey and Jen." I bent down and kissed him on the cheek.

"O.K.," he said smiling. He took a sip of coffee. "Same time...same station?" Remember I love you, Sweet-Love."

"I love you too. I must go now," I answered. "Same time...same station tomorrow. I'll call you tonight." It was all I could do to hold back the tears, but I managed until I got to the car. I bawled like a baby. I felt like I had abandoned my Sweet-Love. I knew he was in good hands but still…so hard being separated after fifty-three years!

I called Peter that night. Our conversation was typical of how we conversed: "Hi, Darling. How's everything?" I queried. "Was dinner good?"

"All right…you're cooking is better," he answered. "Same time…same station?"

"Yes, I'll be there for lunch," I answered back. "Remember I'm in your pocket…sweet dreams, Love. I'll see you tomorrow."

"I love you, Darling," he said. "I'll see you tomorrow."

"Take care of my Darling," I said and hung up the phone. Sadness came over me, but for a moment, as the dogs competed for my attention.

*****

As the months went by, neither of us were happy with Beechwick. There was nothing that kept Peter busy. Most of the time I'd find him in the dining room in the wheelchair fast asleep. Then again we had a terrible time putting up with the Alzheimer's patients. They stole the television remote, the legs to Peter's wheelchair, and a quilt which we got back. They were always wandering in and out of the rooms either because they wanted attention, were bored or confused as to where they were. Granted Peter had dementia, but it was not as bad as the other patients. I felt they should separate the two, but Beechwick wanted to create a feeling of a community.

Thankfully, Peter forgot about escaping, but we found it hard to say goodbye in the afternoons. He always begged me to stay, which made me feel like I was abandoning him. How I wished I could take him home…if only!

Downstairs, the rest of Beechwick was for assisted living. The residents had total independence. I got to know a few. One complaint they had was there was really nothing to do.

*****

Several times I took Lindsey to see Peter during snack time. It was amazing how people responded to her; however, some overshadowed her which made her scared. I would then take her back to Peter. He was overjoyed. When she settled down, I would take her on a one-to-one basis. She adored the attention. I had wanted to take Jen but she was too skittish or high-strung.

One day for lunch I succeeded in taking Peter to The Grille at Westlake. Physical therapy had taught him how to pivot into the passenger's car seat. We were surprised how fast he picked up the technique! At the restaurant guests and staff welcomed us as we found our way to the table. "Beep…beep!" Peter cried out. What a marvelous time we had…it was good to get out in public, and we enjoyed the hearty meal: chicken noodle soup, a ham and cheese omelet with a tossed salad on the side. Peter totally enjoyed himself, in spite of the fact that he was being seen in a wheelchair. Other times, the girls at Beechwick would microwave whatever I would bring in from home. Favorite foods could be a portion of salmon or swordfish I would have the night before, oysters in season, homemade soup, and pitted ripe and green olives. After lunch I'd wheel him back to his room for several Reese's peanut butter cups or York peppermint patties.

A brother of one of the patients came into our room to see Peter's Navy pictures. From that time on my Darling was nicknamed "Lieutenant" around the community. This always brought a broad smile on Peter's face. Moreover, I got Susan, a volunteer, to read to him in the mornings – anything to keep him busy and to help make the time go by. He enjoyed this for a while, until he had a hard time concentrating.

We had a wonderful conversation in his room: I had just finished brushing his teeth and had leaned over giving him a broad hug and a kiss on his cheek. "I love my Darling, my preppy, lawyer Husband...handsome and brave to be putting up with Beechwick." Peter laughed. "I know you don't like it here but the food is good, you live in a lovely suite, and you're loved by the whole staff," I empathized, caressing his shoulders.

"Yes...you're right...I'm lucky that way but I still want to go home," he sighed."Let's go for a walk. I'll prove to you that I can do it." I then took Peter out to the hall and went back to his room to get the walker. Upon my return, he stood right up, grabbed the bars, and walked the length of the unit. I, of course, followed him with the wheelchair.

"Will you look at that?" Patty, an aide, greeted us. "You're doing a fine job!"

We returned to the room. "That was fabulous! I'm proud of you," I reassured him. "Tomorrow, John, the therapist, will be with you. He's certainly doing a good job helping you. I'm proud of you, my Sweet-Darling...oh, I love you."

"That was a workout...I'm tired," he sighed as I massaged his shoulders. "My left shoulder hurts. Don't know why. It throbs...sometimes."

"I'll get the nurse to give you a Tylenol, Sweetheart. Probably the girls are lifting you too hard from the bed, or as you reach for the handicap bar in the bathroom. I'll mention this to the Care Manager. I wish they'd let you have a bedside railing to help you lift up, but evidently it is a New Jersey law that no restraints can be used," I said earnestly.

"You know...you're such a caring wife. I love you, Sweet-Love," he remarked, as he reached for my hand and kissed it. "You're beautiful!"

"I love you too, Darling," I said smiling. I looked at my watch. "It's snack time." We both knew what this meant. We'd have to part.

I placed him at a table in the dining room and went back to the room to collect my things. Returning, Peter had backed up across the room. I apologized to the people at his table. "Did he bump your table?" There was no answer. "You've really pushed yourself backwards, Peter," I laughed.

"I'm in all directions," he stated hesitating between words. "De…men." He was sundowning1

"You have dementia. That's ok. You're having trouble thinking and talking. You'll be seeing the speech therapist in the morning." We were interrupted by the nurse, who gave him his afternoon medications. I asked her for Tylenol, and waited for her to return just to make sure he was given the medication. "That will make you feel better," I reassured him giving him a kiss on the forehead. I should be leaving.

"Ok, but I need my black book, Sweetie," he said emphatically. The book was a kind of a bible to Peter. He used it at the office. It has all sorts of important information, addresses, and so forth.

"I'll bring it in tomorrow…same time...same station. I love you," I said and began to leave. Peter didn't say anything but sipped his coffee.

I met my friend downstairs. I told her about our conversation. We hugged and burst into tears. "I've been there," she sighed. I thanked her for listening and left the building. I sobbed all the way home. Without realizing it, I actually was going through the grieving process of losing a spouse.

At the house, I began having trouble with the dogs as they wouldn't come when called. They were cooped up for too long…somehow I must spend more time with them I told myself…but how?

The next morning Peter met with the speech therapist complaining that the nerve around his mouth wasn't working, and he was having trouble finishing a sentence. She explained to me that the stroke he had in 2008 was making his mouth feel funny. She would increase exercises to three times a day.

As for his shoulder, I took him to the orthopedist who had helped me with my fractured arm. Peter had arthritis, but because he had Parkinson's, he was not a candidate for shoulder replacement surgery. It would be better to put him on a low dose of pain medication and to use heat…if that didn't work then mentholated patches.

I began to see definite changes in my Husband. Still he never complained and was always cheerful…at least he never let the staff know he was uncomfortable. I was the only one he confided in. I eyed the staff like a hawk making sure he was comfortable at all times. I began to feel like they didn't like seeing me every day.

Though nothing was said, their looks made me feel this way. Since the house in New Boston was on the market, I visited Peter through rain, sunshine, sleet or snow! I never missed a day.

Peter developed another problem...during lunch he was trying to feed himself but couldn't reach the spoon to his mouth. In helping him, I discovered he had swallowed four lower teeth that had broken in half. The dentist said that since he wasn't having pain, he wouldn't do anything. A lower denture was not the solution as he had an upper one. Because of Parkinson's disease, there was always a chance of choking.

I commented to Peter, "I don't understand. We've nursed your lower teeth with mouthwash and brushing. I guess it's because the nurse gives you medication with yogurt or a watered-down sugary drink six times a day without rinsing...or the medications alone can cause tooth decay!"

"I'll be all right, Sweet-Love," he responded proudly. "Don't worry I can chew." I laughed.

"I've just been fitted with a bridge and you have a denture. You and I have always had problems with our teeth. To think of the misery you went through with the implants that didn't take because of bone loss. That was in Houston," I remarked. "You let me know if you ever have pain, please." I kissed him on the cheek.

"I will, Sweet-Love. The girls don't like you to complain," he sighed. "That's why I smile all the time."

"Well, you can complain to me, Darling...any time," I reassured him wearing a broad grin. "That's because I love you."

The physical therapist interrupted us. He had gotten the walker from Peter's room. "Let's take a walk," he said."Ceci, you can follow us with the wheelchair." I nodded "yes." But Peter couldn't get up. He tried but rigidity stood in the way. John finished the session by doing leg and arm exercises. I thanked John and gave Peter a strong hug. Looking into his hazel eyes I said smiling, "I'm proud of you my sweet, handsome Husband...you gave it all you could...but you mustn't give up. It's just a bad day. Tomorrow will be a better day."

"I love you. You're a beautiful princess," he said.

"I don't know about that!" I laughed and kissed him on his lips. "My do I love, love, love you, my handsome Prince. I'm proud of you in every way. You're a brilliant lawyer...look at the way you drew up the real estate papers with the lawyer in Great Barrington over the right-of-way to "Thurtilperk Hill"...when we no longer had to drive over the meadow but were able to have a road built to the house...you're a devoted father, and oh, what a preppy, handsome Husband you are...you always put me first...you made me feel loved." Peter's eyes lit up.

"I feel better. Can I have a cup of coffee?" he asked. With that I wheeled him into the dining room. It was snack time and we had to part, but he didn't seem to mind.

"I'll call you tonight, Sweetheart," I said.

"Ok," he responded and sipped his coffee.

*****

For the past two months I've seen Peter go downhill. It was all over Beechwick before I knew it – he now needed two girls to get him dressed and to use the bathroom. He no longer could use a television remote or dial a phone, needed to be fed, forgot how to use a wheelchair, and had no interest in anything except being with his Spoose! It was our strong love that kept us close. We adored each other. We had become soul mates.

One day I found Peter totally confused, half asleep, sitting in the dining room. He couldn't make a bit of sense. I spoke to the nurse, who took his blood pressure discovering that it was 78/35. The cardiologist had told me that he had fluctuating blood pressure…to give him salt in a glass of water if it got low. This I did. Within a few minutes Peter was back to normal. The nurse called the cardiologist, upon my request, and was told to take him off of Zocor. I blame Sinemet, which lowers blood pressure, a serious side effect.

We kept our appointment with the neurologist who asked Peter many questions which he was not able to answer. He had a hard time communicating. She diagnosed aphasia. According to the National Aphasia Association: "Aphasia impairs the ability to speak and understand others, and most people with aphasia experience difficulty reading and writing. It is an acquired communication disorder that impairs a person's ability to process language but does not affect intelligence."

Soon after, we returned to Beechwick in time for lunch. Peter ate like a horse. I had brought in liverwurst and green pitted olives which he devoured quickly. We then went outside to the garden and sat in the shade for a half hour. I encouraged him to talk more for exercise. I also talked about his 80$^{th}$ birthday coming up on September 15, 2011, but he was no help in that respect. As I took him back to his room to do his teeth, he said, "You stimulate me!"

"You said you wanted to treat me like a princess when we get to Heaven," I responded. "Well, I'm going to treat you like a prince when we get there, Sweetheart. Yesterday you scared me the way you acted- not talking, spilling food, not cooperating, and refusing to stand up." Peter was deep in thought.

"I love you, Sweet-Love," he sighed as he tried to get the words out.

"That's all right, Darling," I assured him trying to be upbeat. "We love each other. That's all that matters." I knew he couldn't help it…sometimes his mind won't let him talk, sit, stand or walk. What got me through this, day after day, was resilience. I was now aware of the situation. As Parkinson's progressed, I was able to go forward.

We celebrated Peter's birthday by having lunch in Beechwick's assisted living dining room. I had invited my brother, Mike; his lovely German wife, Babette; my sister, Barbara; and Sharon to help us celebrate. After consulting each one as to what he or she wanted to eat, I picked up the food at a fine Japanese restaurant. Peter was flabbergasted when I wheeled him into the room. He had such a twinkle in his eyes and he held an incredible grin on his face, which I will never forget. We had such a good time with lots of laughter. Much to my surprise, Beechwick went out of their way providing drinks, coffee and tea, and presented Peter with a small decorated birthday cake. It was a good day for my Husband. I hadn't seen him laugh as hard as he had for a long, long time!

On Christmas weekend we celebrated with an afternoon visit from Mike, Babette, Barbara, and Sharon. Family support was extremely important now, especially for Peter. I was thankful that they began to visit more often. We did see Sharon, of course, most weekends, work permitting!

*****

In February, 2012, Peter needed to go to the bathroom during lunch. Two girls took him to his room. After fifteen minutes they hadn't returned. Instead, I went to them. I found my Husband on the bedroom floor. His bed had been pushed over by the window, and the lamp on the floor was broken. To this day I don't know what happened; however, I refused to let them take him to the hospital, as he said he was all right. Beechwick confined him to the bed. He was not allowed to sit in a chair. As a result, while Peter was napping, I slipped out of the facility and went to Hawthorne Grove Rehabilitation and Skilled Nursing. I arranged to have Peter transferred as soon as possible; consequently, upon informing the Supervisor of Beechwick, I was told I had to give thirty days' notice. I responded by saying "You can't expect him to lie in one position in bed for that length of time. I'll sue you. We're going to Hawthorne." Peter, thus, was transferred immediately by ambulance to the nursing home – there he entered an unusually cheerful and compassionate kind of life, an entirely different way of joyful living.

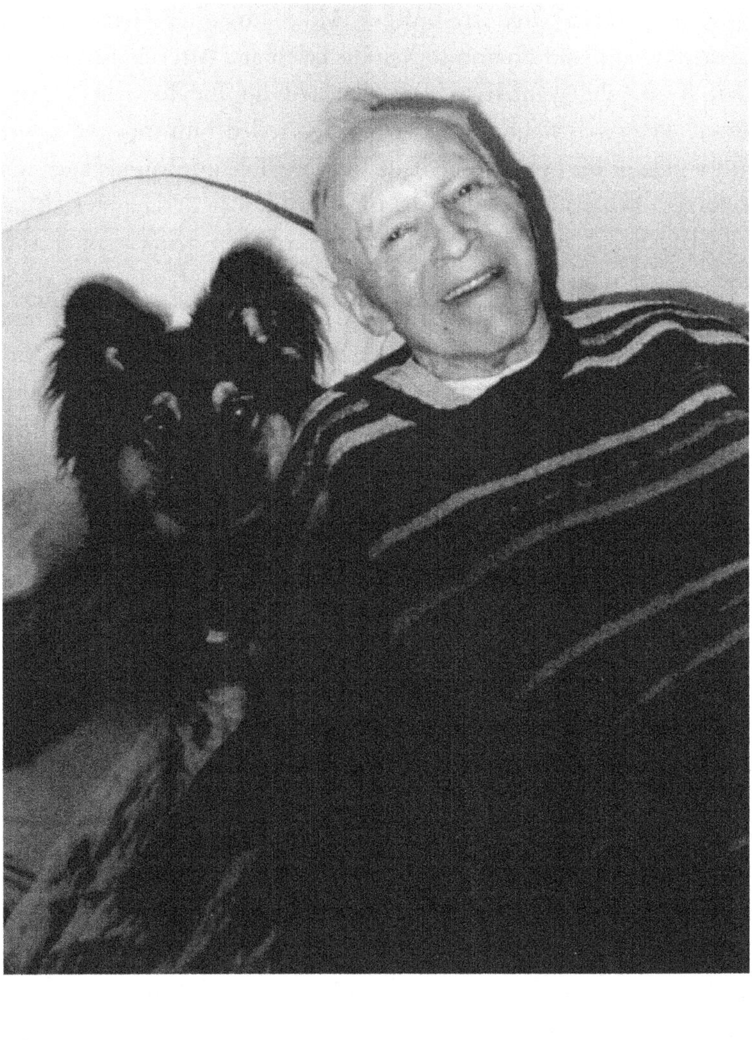

Peter and Jen

# Part Seven: Acceptance

## An Unexpected Move

I met Peter at Hawthorne just as he was being taken out of the ambulance. I thanked the driver and wheeled him down the hall to his room passing the large glass windowed Day Room. "I go in there?" Peter sighed with trepidation. "Just sit…a waste of time!"

"No…no, Sweetheart. That is where you have meals," I said being upbeat. I tried to be encouraging and reassuring as much as possible. From that day on, I was determined to make him happy by participating in as many activities each day if offered. Thankfully, I was able to order lunch for $3.00, which we had in his room. His roommate, nicknamed "Junior," was an engaging and attractive man who had had a stroke. His wife, Colleen, was fun to be around. We all got along famously. We were lucky!

The Head Nurse and various members of the staff came into the room introducing themselves. They were charming and extremely friendly. Peter found himself laughing. I could see him begin to relax. Emma would be his regular Aide…pleasant and knowledgeable, having been at Hawthorne for sixteen years. I explained to her about rigidity. She knew all about it. "We live each day to the fullest with encouragement and hope. In the beginning he will have physical, speech and occupational therapies," she said. "Everyone here is special."

While Emma tucked Peter in for a nap, I returned to Beechwick to clean out his room. With the help of several friends, we removed the furniture and clothes. How happy I was to get out of there!

Upon returning to Hawthorne, just as the 3 o'clock shift had arrived, Peter and I met Joe, an orderly, who would be taking care of him and would call each night before Peter went to sleep. This routine was a marvelous way of communicating. It kept us incredibly close. After a nap, Joe helped Peter into the wheelchair, where upon we toured the whole facility. There was a large activity room, the attractive lobby where patients and families congregated, several outside gardens, and in one wing a snack bar offering cookies and drinks. On Peter's floor ice cream was offered each afternoon. We looked forward to tomorrow, Wednesday, when there would be live entertainment after lunch. As we returned to the room, I picked up a chocolate ice cream cup and a container of cranberry juice.

"What do you think, Darling?" I asked enthusiastically on the way. "Hawthorne is certainly an improvement over Beechwick. You'll be happy here."

"Sweetie, Joe…I like him," Peter said smiling which in turn made me smile.

"I do too," I agreed. "Hi, Junior…Colleen." They were watching television. Much to our surprise, my two friends had brought in the extra bureau and had unpacked the clothing, while we were scouting the nursing home. I thanked them and fed Peter the ice cream. Colleen told us about her husband, who was busy watching "Animal Planet." Junior spoke very little. He was paralyzed on the left side, having no use of his arm or leg…he had been at Hawthorne for two years. As it turned out in the long run, he and Peter got along well, according to Joe. I was relieved.

At four o'clock, I wheeled Peter into the Day Room where he would have to wait for dinner. Joe would feed him.

"I'll be leaving now, Sweetheart," I said and kissed him on the cheek. I love my Darling."

"I'll call you," Peter replied, looking into my sparkling blue eyes. "You're beautiful."

"Why thank you, Sweet-Love…same time…same station tomorrow," I said to reassure him. "I love you. Talk to you tonight."

"Ok," he answered. I could hear in the background, as I walked toward the lobby, Peter being introduced to the other patients. I felt happy for a moment, but sadness came over me. There was the usual emptiness I always felt leaving my precious Husband. I cried in the car.

That night Joe called giving the phone receiver to Peter. "Hi, Darling, have a good night…sweet dreams. I love you," I emphasized.

"Good night, Darling…I love you," he responded. "Joe, where are you?" There was silence. I hung up feeling extremely sad. It was hard knowing that I was gradually losing my Husband. At least Peter is in a better place. He was in good hands I told myself, but I must take better care of myself. I need more rest. That night I spent a lot of time with Lindsey and Jen, and was tucked in at nine o'clock.

The next day I arrived in time for lunch, which gave me an extra hour of sleep that morning. I ordered meals for the rest of the week as we would eat in the Day Room. It was easier and more convenient for me…also, one way of getting to know the other patients and members of their families, if they ever came!

As I entered the Day Room and looked around, I greeted the patients. "Hi, ladies!" I then walked over to my sleeping Husband sitting in his wheelchair at a table, and kissed him on the forehead. He was overjoyed to see me. He had the biggest smile on his face. Each day I did this. I began to converse with the patients individually, which was fun. By offering Peter a cup of water signaled the beginning of friendships! Everyone wanted water, which I graciously handed out from the water cooler around the corner from the Day Room.

After lunch on Peter's second day at the nursing home, on a Wednesday, I wheeled him into the large Activity Room. There we sat at the back of the room behind all the assisted and nursing home patients seated in rows. We were entertained by a marvelous couple...the wife sang Broadway songs while the husband played various instruments. All the while, Peter and I held hands, enjoying every minute of the cheerful, familiar music. He would stare at me and whisper, "You're beautiful or I love you." Music was instrumental in helping Peter with Parkinson's. He would forget the pain and tingling for a while. Although he was sundowning, he seemed more alert, especially having his Sweetie-Spoose by his side. Our holding hands exemplified our love for each other. Also, it was a way of communicating if his aphasia took over at the time. I'm told that touch and praise are very important in reaching out to a dementia person...as is direct eye contact, by simply smiling and looking into Peter's eyes saying "I love you"...or complimenting and reminiscing. Every day I tried all these, which made Peter feel loved, happy, and relaxed. In turn, he made me feel loved and appreciated.

Physical therapy excused my Darling. His rigidity wouldn't allow him to stand up, much less take a step. Speech exercises helped immensely, depending upon whether it was a good or bad day. With occupational therapy he was given helpful tools to use, such as a deep, rounded, curved plate for his finely ground food. The former helped him with chewing, the plate from spilling. All and all Hawthorne got us through each day always making sure Peter was comfortable.

Every afternoon we met the same family members, taking care of their spouses, as I was, in the lobby where we sat and conversed. I was amazed that only a handful of family members appeared. Some of the patients I spoke to missed their loved ones. It was extremely sad for I knew how happy Peter was when I appeared at a certain time of day. He could count on me. It gave him a feeling of being loved and not forgotten. He could trust me.

# The Quagmire of Dementia

Some days Peter couldn't speak at all or he'd blurt out with sharp remarks. Others, he'd talk up a storm. I yearned for the latter.

We kept our appointment with our neurologist in Freehold. She put my Husband through a series of tests including having a CAT scan. The x-ray showed a darkening of the right side of his brain which showed deterioration. In one of the tests the highest score was thirty. Peter was eleven. My heart sank. I wanted to cry…no wonder he was having trouble. On top of that, he felt a constant tingling in his body due to rigidity. The doctor said, under the circumstances, he was doing well because I was taking care of him. At this stage of life, he needed all the love I could give him, especially recalling past memories, if at all possible. I thanked the doctor who adjusted Peter's Sinemet by giving him a prescription for two at seven am, two at one pm, and two at dinner. At times he would freeze as the medication began to wear off. This change in doses helped enormously, not only by making him more alert and responsive, but aided Hawthorne's staff in handling him.

As I write from my journal: "When we are in his room, or in the Lobby, enjoying rest after we had finished our walk, I'd bring up past memories of things we did together – our wedding, his proposal, receiving Sharon at The Adoption Agency, Bermuda, and his trips to India. I'll hug him and tell him I miss snuggling in bed, just to be near him. This takes him out of his shell. He said he slept so well last night as I had told him I was in his arms…the day before we had sundaes…the entire Hawthorne…the first banana split I had had in forty years. It was delicious and energizing!"

"In early May of 2012, I, with the two dogs, went up to New Boston for nine days – so hard not having Peter around – so many memories. WEMCO, the electric company, came at 7:45 am to check ruts they had made with their truck in the yard. If Peter had been here, he would have thrown on his pants and greeted the man. I was out of my brace. Have a terrible time on the phone with him am and pm."

The house is still on the market. Have had two offers but declined them because they were too low; however, there was a gentleman, a novelist, who fell in love with the property, remarking, "It's so romantic!" He decided not to buy because of the price. The best part of being up here is for the dogs. How they love to run around exploring, without being confined by an invisible fence…no porcupines or bears this time, thank goodness! I had a terrible time with Peter on the phone morning and evening. His mind wanders. "Collecting my thoughts," he would say. He was unable to hold the phone receiver this time. "Say hello," Joe said. "Say, Honey, I love you," I responded by saying, "I love my Darling…I'm in your arms…sweet dreams." "Goodnight, Love," he mumbled. Tomorrow will be different I tell myself. Maybe it will be a better day for my Sweetheart.

Peter was overjoyed to see me upon my return from New Boston. Joe had taken good care of him. Colleen asked me to feed my Husband at lunch, as the morning aide was feeding him too fast with enormous bites. He could easily choke. I said I would. It seemed that when I enjoyed a sandwich I had brought in from home, Peter would try to feed himself. I told him I had had a dream that he asked me to marry him. He wore a broad smile on his face. I caressed his cheek with my hand and said, "I do love you, Mr. Hitchcock. His response surprised me. "I love you too, Mrs. Hitchcock."

After lunch we went into the Activity Room to play games. Peter came in third place in one. We then participated in the sing-a-long where someone would play the piano, while the residents would sing the songs. It was fun. Other times there were movies in the afternoons, get togethers for special treats, such as milk shakes, ice cream cones, large pretzels with nonalcoholic O'Doul's, or cookies and sundaes…on Wednesday's entertainment, and one particular game I liked was "What would you do?" The residents would play the part of the lawyer after being given a case. At first Peter tried to be the lawyer, but some of the cases were too hard. Peter lost interest. We enjoyed the nondenominational religious service each Sunday morning.

As the weather warmed up, we'd spend a great deal of time outside. I'd wheel him around Hawthorne which was a hike. Usually we'd end up in the garden joining Junior and Colleen. There we met familiar faces of family members with their spouses soaking up the warm, bright sunshine.

On Flag Day we were in Peter's room, just about to celebrate in the Activity Room, when Peter blurted out, "You're beautiful…love you." I kissed him on the lips in return whispering, "Thank you…I love you too." I never knew what he'd come out and say. But certainly I knew he loved me, which made me feel good and appreciated. Colleen and I wheeled our spouses to the Activity Room. There Peter bellowed out voluntarily the French Anthem, much to everyone's surprise. "Wow…I'm proud of you, Sweetheart," I said. I was told by Junior that some nights he would speak out loud in French while dreaming!

One day we had a conversation, which makes me chuckle as I write. Peter was staring at me in a loving way. "I like you," he said. My reaction was, "LIKE…what about LOVE?" I asked. He laughed so hard, which in turn made me laugh. Tears were running down our faces. "You are something," I chuckled.

"I like you too. But you had better say 'I love you' or I won't come back tomorrow!"

"I love you," he giggled. "Sweet-Love."

"That's better, Sweetheart," I joked. That night in our phone conversation I kidded him, "I like you, Sweetheart." He laughed and said, "Goodnight, Darling."

The next day I brought in several picture books from his collection. One was of London, where he had been stationed in the Navy for two years. He had fun flipping through the pages. "Tomorrow I'll bring in a photo album of pictures of when we first met. Edie and Alan are in them too. He was your roommate at Columbia Law School, and my friend, Edith Bailey, at St. Luke's," I said. Peter couldn't remember who they were. I told him about their wedding. He was best man while I was the maid of honor. They lived right next to our apartment at 133 West 12$^{th}$ Street in New York City. He nodded "no," giving me a strange look. He was having a hard time communicating with me…so hard. Tomorrow he'll probably remember.

*****

Peter began to have severe pain in his left shoulder where he had arthritis. I was told it took three girls to remove him from the toilet. He wouldn't, or couldn't, pull up on the bar. Physical therapy was called in and ok'd a Hoyer lift. They don't like to use it because the patient will never stand up again. I argued, " He can't stand anyway. Besides using it would save his shoulder." Peter was miserable. Tylenol with Codeine was ordered. I asked them to give one early in the morning after breakfast, before I was to arrive or he would sleep through lunch and my visit...to use the mentholated patch in the afternoon and again the dosage before going to bed. This plan worked out well, thank goodness.

Peter's rigidity got worse in the early morning. Sometimes his whole body would shake…as though he would flip out of bed. I witnessed this one day while he was in the wheelchair. It scared me. "What was that?" he'd ask me. "I don't know except the rigidity…you'll be ok. It doesn't happen very often," I said trying to be upbeat. That night in our phone conversation, he seemed depressed. I assured him I'd be there tomorrow same time…same station. "Thank God you're here. I love you, Darling," he replied.

From my journal: "July 10 – Tuesday 2012…I haven't written because Peter is going downhill – that is, he lacks emotion most of the time. I hold his hand when we are entertained with music. He is more aware and loving."

"At lunch now when he doesn't want something he turns his head away or he tightens his mouth – not often but hard to feed him when it happens. He is quieter now and says very little. I wonder if he can.

When I ask questions, he won't answer – unless I say I'm going home if he sleeps. Yet, when he talks to me over the phone, he will say 'Yes please,' if I say I'm in his arms. Too many medications (29). He still surprises me with what he says sometimes – perhaps a joke in French?"

"I feel so alone and want to totally hug him but he seems so cold sometimes – his attention span is short. On the phone he says a few things, then asks for Joe. I do most of the talking, or we can be watching a good movie...he wants to leave...always we must keep moving...take walks...change the scenery."

"Friday the 13th was a good time with Peter. He was so open and loving after lunch in his room. I was watching "Animal Planet" on television, after doing his teeth (which is never done in the facility, by the way...just rinsing at night. Most residents have many teeth missing!) Peter would follow me around. When I sat on the bed, he smiled at me saying, 'You're my Sweetie-Spoose. I love you.' I was surprised. We stared at each other, and then I kissed him on the lips. 'I love you. You're my Darling,' I said. Peter reached for my hand saying, 'you're beautiful.'"

There was still that powerful chemistry between the two of us...we were connected to each other, soul mates.

# Just You and Me

On September the 12th, 2012, I returned to New Boston with Lindsey and Jen to have the cottage winterized and to take the property off the market. Carol Riiska met me as I pulled into the circular driveway. What a good friend she was. She unpacked the car, visited for a while, and later took off for home.

I was extremely tired that night after five hours of driving bumper to bumper on the states' highways. I climbed into bed early, after talking to Peter on the phone, and realized I hadn't taken Coumadin, a blood thinner, which was important because I had a pacemaker. I immediately hopped out of bed, grabbed the walker, for I was out of brace, and marched into the dining room. In reaching for the medication on the table, I grabbed the top of the chair for support, which in turn toppled the chair. I buckled, falling backwards landing on my buttocks and lower spine. To make a long story short, Carol returned the next morning, took the dogs to a kennel in Great Barrington, while I was being transported by ambulance to the hospital there. I had severely injured my spine, having two compression fractures, bulging disks, and a herniated disk. Thankfully, no osteoporosis, but I had stenosis, a narrowing of the spine. After a week, I was taken by ambulance to Birchwood for rehabilitation, and then onto Hawthorne in Jackson for more physical therapy. Carol arranged the winterization of the house with the help of our dear friend and handyman, Steve Kopiec.

It was my idea to be transferred, as I would be able to see Peter every day. But I had one problem...I was told not to push his wheelchair. It was incredibly wonderful to be with my Love between my sessions of physical therapy. Thankfully, the aides voluntarily helped me. It was quite a trek to his wing – great exercise. As a result, I lost ten pounds. We couldn't have meals together, but I managed to see my Husband in the afternoons, after our naps, and in the late evenings. Peter and I enjoyed every minute of our being together.

Steve drove Lindsey and Jen down in the Honda Odyssey. He was met by our friend, Joy Farrar, who took him to the bus station and then brought the dogs to us for a visit. I don't know what I would have done had I not had Carol, Steve, and Joy to help me! Lindsey and Jen were happy to see us, but were confused, as they would again be taken to a kennel in Jackson until I was able to leave Hawthorne. As I write this, the accident was a total disaster in every way...certainly changing my way of living by slowing me down. Needless to say, sometimes I felt like kicking myself!

With Joy's help, I returned to the Jackson house soon after. How wonderful it was to be home once again with my dogs. I immediately began my visits every day to Hawthorne after sessions of Decompression at The Spine Institute each morning, which helped a lot along with an epidural injection.

I write from my journal: "With sundowning Peter makes more sense – can talk so much better – is more restless and involved with things around him. At night he's so loving – sometimes you'd never know he had Parkinson's."

"Last week Peter finished lunch after being fed. Rigidity bounced him from a sitting into a lying position. It took four aides to put him into a geriatric chair – I was shocked and, needless to say, horrified. He has since been in and out of his wheelchair. A week later, I had the leg rests extended. He hasn't been in a geriatric chair since. I am having trouble getting him to talk, much less trying to understand – yet he expresses himself when he sundowns. He has no interest in television – loves the musical programs, though at first doesn't want to go."

"We talk about Heaven. I tell him I am proud of him the way he is handling Parkinson's. 'Just think when we said our vows – for richer or poorer, in sickness and in health, 'til death do us part.' Peter interrupted by laughing which in turn made me laugh. It's good to be able to talk about death. Things are happening in our bodies because of our ages. 'Peter you're almost 81 – I'm almost there!' 'How about that,' he said."

"January 2013, Joe remarked as he was putting him on the Hoyer lift, 'He doesn't know what he's doing – he's indifferent!' For the first time I'm realizing Peter isn't with it – whether it's the Tylenol with Codeine three times a day to stop the shoulder pain or dementia! I'm tired of the silence between the two of us. He won't talk, yet at night, if I tell him I love him, he will respond by telling me he loves me. This certainly has upset me."

"Now, I'm beginning to realize that dementia has really set in, which is a blessing – he doesn't know what's going on – or does he – that's Parkinson's. His Long Term Care ends 11/30/13. Can I bring him home? I can't lift him, and I can't stand the idea of having a live-in. Tomorrow I see our financial advisor to discuss how we can afford the nursing home at $10,000 a month. Surely we are going to run out of money. I feel so alone. I've already lost my two loves: Penny and Meghan, our dogs (our grandchildren as Peter called them) and now Peter."

"I got the bad news from John that we must sell the New Boston house. After Joe called me one night, Peter wanted to call again. 'I love you, Sweetie. It's just you and me,' he said. 'I miss you so much,' I replied. 'I'm watching television, then I'll go to bed. It's a strange world without you here.' 'You can say that again,' answered Peter. 'I'll dream about you if you will dream about me,' I said. 'Yes please,' he exclaimed. 'Good night, Darling. Just you and me!'"

"He surprised me one day after I had taken him for a walk, when I asked him if he'd like to take a nap. 'It's better than being here.' – depression? What can I do to make him happier? I then began to plan on taking Peter home in November. There was no reaction when I mentioned this to my Love. In fact, he wasn't a bit interested and didn't want to leave Hawthorne."

"On February12, 2013, I felt like celebrating our fifty-fourth year together. Peter had no feelings. During entertainment he didn't want to hold hands – just sleep. This afternoon he was sundowning in his geriatric chair, which he hated, calling out 'hello' many times and trying to stretch and get out of the chair. I was ready to go home, had put on my coat, and kissed him goodbye. He grabbed my hand so hard it hurt. He grabbed my clothing, his clothing. He wouldn't listen to my cry. To me he was going berserk! I took him to the Day Room – he continued to grab whatever he could – no emotion – just far away. How can I bring him home? On my way out of the Day Room I asked the Head Nurse to give him something – perhaps lower the pain medicine."

"Peter isn't eating much anymore. He doesn't draw on a straw, so we're using cups. I don't dare use Listerine. He swallows the toothpaste. I was able to put my check against his and whispered how much I love him. 'Did you enjoy the music?' I asked. 'Oh, yes,' he answered. 'I wish we could have danced,' I said smiling. I kissed him on the cheek. The aide then put him down for a nap. 'He would stay in bed for dinner,' she said. I left Peter sleeping and went to the Day Room after ordering his favorite cheese omelet, cottage cheese, and sherbet. I had a delightful chat with my resident friends. We talked about the music. 'I cried,' said Marie, ninety-four years old. 'It brought back so many memories. You know we loved each other so much.' 'How's your back,' asked the sixty-five year old. I told her the epidural injection helped but I was sore. 'How about Peter?' she asked. 'He's asleep now so I'm going home. You know we love each other,' I said. 'He isn't doing well. We talk about Heaven. He tells me he is going to treat me like a princess when we get to Heaven. I will treat him like a prince.' I looked at Marie, the ninety-four year old and said, 'Your prince is looking down on you!'"

"Marie said, 'You have such a spark in your eyes. You're so cheerful, Ceci. There's a way about you. There's something you have that makes us happy and gives us hope.' 'Well,' I said. 'You're going to make me cry.' I changed the subject by talking about the dogs. 'You light up everything,' said Marie as she squeezed my hand."

'Thank you…I wish things were different with Peter," I said. I kissed her on the cheek. 'Well, you all have a good night. I'll see you tomorrow.' I cried in the car going home – I miss Peter so much."

"Easter Sunday, like yesterday afternoon, Peter hadn't eaten much during the day. He's down to 147 lbs. from 163 in one month – and he's quite an eater. He's having trouble with swallowing. Uses Boost or skim milk to wash down food."

"Sharon came – it was so great to have her. She, too, is aware of how things have changed. She helped me feed Peter - he closes his mouth tight if he doesn't want food. I asked him if it hurt swallowing. 'You're not feeling well, are you?' I asked rubbing his neck. 'No,' he responded. 'But...' I continued, 'you need to keep up your strength. You have to eat something even if it is just liquid – I love my Darling.' I caressed his face. 'I want to make you comfortable. Parkinson's is for the pits – I hate to see you suffer. Please take care of yourself for me – you're my whole life but it's o.k. to let go – we'll meet each other later.' 'Happy Easter, Darling. I love you,' he mumbled."

"Tomorrow I'll talk to Hospice to see what is involved. I feel he is doing this intentionally by not eating because Long Term Care ends soon. He wants to make sure I will be taken care of in the future. He always puts me first; however, he's not used to lying and wasting time in a geriatric chair. He's miserable and his quality of life is terrible. He can't read – sleeping passes the time. But when he sees me, there is that rewarding smile – a smile everyone comments on. My Sweet-Love once told me, 'You have to smile even if you don't want to. You have to look happy or they get upset.' That makes me sad. 'Sometimes when you smile, that means you're strong,' I told him."

The day after Easter (Monday, April 1, 2013) Peter was put on Hospice. We were introduced to the Chaplain, the director and two aides, who would alternate taking care of him. "Peter has lost so much weight in a month. 'You're on strike,' I kid him – his spirits are high with me but will only touch fluids using a cup – last night he kept telling me that he loved me over and over again."

"The people in Hospice are wonderful, kind, and compassionate. The Chaplain said several prayers for us – 'The Lord is My Shepherd' and 'The Lord's Prayer.' She will bring communion soon, which we would love. The new geriatric chair arrived and they're giving me a geriatric wheelchair that I can push to take him outside when the weather gets warmer. They've reduced his pills, and he is shaking less – a miracle – on Codeine but not Morphine yet. He is having indigestion so I try to give him extra ice cream in the afternoon – eggs, two bowls of soup, yogurt and sherbet at night along with a Boost. The sixth of April – Saturday – Gaylord is here from Hawaii. He recently moved there."

"In the Lobby, while chatting with Gaylord, we notice that Peter was breathing quickly – rapidly. I took him to his room and oxygen was administered. Throughout the rest of the afternoon he was much more comfortable – also told me he loved me over and over again, when we hugged. That night the phone conversation was the same. It was wonderful. 'I love you, Darling,' he said. 'Have a good night, sweet dreams. I'll see you same time…same station tomorrow. I love you, Darling,' I replied and hung up."

There was a dispute over funeral arrangements among family members. Sharon said no funeral home/chapel – Gaylord – church only-reception at home. I solved it by asking Peter. He said he would like a church funeral. Gaylord, in the meantime, went to the Episcopal Church of St. Uriel the Archangel in Sea Girt, New Jersey. He knew the minister well. The next morning I did visit the church, which was as beautiful, as Gaylord said. I wondered if people would make the trip. I was given a tour and met Father Griffin, who said he would be available anytime night or day to give Peter Last Rites – so thoughtful – such a kind and compassionate man. He came to Hawthorne many times, always offering communion. On one visit he tried to talk to Peter who couldn't speak; however, I was sure my Husband listened intensely to Father's words."

"One night; however, I spoke to my Darling on the phone for the first time in a long time. He was passionate, concerned, and told me he loved me over and over."

"Hospice has been wonderful in taking care of Peter. He continues not to want to eat, is losing weight, and most of the time can't speak except when sundowning – he now mumbles, though – saying 'thank you,' 'yes' or 'you've got that right.' Some days he stares (every other day). It scares me. Hospice says it is a Level of Dying – he is thinking of the past, his friends, and his marriage."

"The next day I visited the funeral home making arrangements. We will have TAPS. Peter was happy when I mentioned this – that it would be played at the end of the service. His eyes lit up and he had that broad smile on his face which in turn made me smile. 'I love you, Darling' I told him."

"Eventually, Peter developed a horrible cough, which I'm sure must have scared him. Knowing him all these years, he hated to cough, much less get a cold, or be around anyone who coughs." He refused food, also medications, which had to be crushed and put in cranberry juice with a thickener. What he ate or drank went down into his lungs. Hospice is now keeping him in bed to rest making him as comfortable as possible. They have given me CD's to play which Peter loved. "Camelot" was his favorite."

"The night before he died, Joe, our favorite aide, called as usual to say goodnight. Peter couldn't talk. I speak and tell him I love him, see him same time…same station tomorrow, sweet dreams. I'm in his arms and that I love him – 'you're my Sweetie-Man –have a good night.' With that he mumbled loud noises and wouldn't stop. He was telling me that he wanted something. I told him I'd call the Head Nurse. He stopped – no noise – I said, 'Sweet dreams, Darling. I love you.' He started up again – his cough was bad. I told him I'd ask the nurse to give him Morphine for the pain. I then hung up."

"I did call the nurse. From his room, she said she had given him Morphine under his tongue. Hospice called me several hours later. 'Your Husband is resting peacefully. We're taking care of him – get some sleep.'"

"On May 14, 2013, the morning nurse called me asking me to get to Hawthorne – call family members, and that Hospice has been with him all morning, the Chaplain saying prayers."

"I got there as fast as I could. I think Peter was trying to tell me that he was dying and to please come in last night. I found him in an unbelievable situation, surrounded by Hospice members saying prayers – his eyes sunken, his body cold, so very much near the end. I said, 'Hi, Sweetheart.' I leaned over and gave him a hug and rested my head on his shoulders. I whispered, 'Remember you're going to treat me like a Princess when we get together, and you'll be my Prince. I wonder if Heaven has a Princess and a Prince. You go now, and I'll follow you, my Darling. I love you, Peter – you're the best Husband and Father. You've been so brave Sweetheart – now it's time to rest – no more Parkinson's. Sharon is coming any minute. She loves you so much – you've been such a great Dad – remember Daddy-Daughter walks – I'm so proud of you, Sweetheart. I love you, Peter.' I hugged him with my head on his chest – 'Just you and me. I love you, I love you, Peter – stay with me, be with me, and watch over me – you're the love of my life.' Peter took his last breath and died. It was as though he was waiting for me before he let go. 'My Darling, you are in a better place now,' I said out loud, kissing him on the forehead."

While this was happening, Mike, my brother, his wife, Babette, and Joy had been in the room the whole time. It was comforting to have them. The nurse gave me his wedding band, which I wear with my wedding rings, having never taken them off since that day. Sharon arrived too late even though I had spent over $200.00 to get her to Hawthorne by taxi from Brooklyn. She was devastated. In a way, I'm glad she wasn't there for his appearance and silence would have upset her immensely. Ironically, when I arrived earlier that morning, the dark rolling clouds in the sky looked like they would burst into flooding rain, but later when we all walked to our cars, there was bright sunshine, the sky clear blue, with not a cloud in sight. To me that was a sign that Peter was with me. "Just you and me," I whispered as my eyes welled with tears.

# Epilogue: Reaching Out

It was a warm, sunny morning on Saturday, May 25, 2013, when I arrived early before the Memorial Service at eleven o'clock in honor of my Husband, Lt. Peter Tilden Hitchcock. I placed a Navy portrait of him on a stand in the front hall of the Episcopal Church of St. Uriel the Archangel in Sea Girt, New Jersey, where people would notice it as they walked in the door. The rest of the photographs, portraying Peter's life of eighty-one years, were placed on a table in Hulbert Hall.

I was surprised, and overjoyed to be able to welcome thirty-six guests. They came to celebrate Peter's life with me…friends, neighbors, and family members, including three children. Father Gaylord Hitchcock and Father Russell Griffin had created a beautiful service – a Mass of Christian Burial, which included Peter's favorite "Battle Hymn of the Republic" and several others he had asked for.

Gaylord gave the Homily – a wonderful tribute to his brother, Peter. Following was the Liturgy of the Eucharist, where we sang "The Lord's Prayer." Tears welled in my eyes as I thought back to the time the two of us sang the Hymn on Sunday mornings at church. Then again I tried to hide my sadness, but with little success, as "Amazing Grace" was being played. I said to myself, "Oh, do I wish you were with me, Peter." Immediately, I felt his presence and heard an inner voice, "I'm right here, Sweet-Love." A sudden peace came over me. Tears were replaced by a feeling of pride. I visualized Peter beaming when a U. S. Military bugler trumpeted TAPS from outside the front of the Church of St. Uriel. It was an honor to be Lieutenant, Senior Grade, Peter Tilden Hitchcock's wife, especially so when the U. S. Military presented the newly folded American flag.

I received many, many compliments over the Service and luncheon I had had catered and served in Hulbert Hall. It was an amazing feeling receiving such support from all those that attended. They, too, loved Peter.

It has been an incredible journey for me writing "Same Time…Same Station." I have enjoyed every minute of it. Not only has it been therapeutic, but it has kept me close to my Husband. Though at times it hasn't been easy, I am proud, at eighty-one, of what I have written. I hope my words have been inspiring and uplifting. Peter, feeling our relationship as Husband and Wife was special, wanted me to write about our strong love and compassion we shared – to include our love letters written during our courtship and marriage. They kept us close when we were apart. He was extremely upset that even though advancements have been made to prevent the symptoms of his Disease, Parkinson's cannot be stopped. He always had hoped that one day research would stop his rigidity from progressing. To think that my Grandfather, William Starr Myers, had it in the 1950's…very little has changed.

Peter also wanted to call attention to those who have been diagnosed with Parkinson's…that it is not a death sentence. He had it for twenty-six years, going back to the late 1980's, when he was flicking the two fingers on his left hand, off and on. He was a successful lawyer for thirty-seven years, a loving Father, and a devoted Husband…an avid history buff, a compassionate friend, always having a positive outlook rather than worrying about the future. Our early retirement years were full of love, joy, laughter, and all the adventures at "Thurtilperk Hill," our ninety-two-year-old seasonal home in New Boston in the Berkshires. Don't let the diagnosis of Parkinson's get you down, but instead go forward, have fun, do something new. We all are born with a gift of some sort – use it – loving every minute of every day enjoying life to its fullest. We don't know what tomorrow will bring, but rarely does one die from Parkinson's. Peter was an exception as dementia and rigidity took over. Usually, heart disease gets you first.

I learned one thing visiting my friends at Hawthorne. Patients feel it is the end of the road and wait for death. I quote an excerpt from a letter of my Aunt Nelle's, wife of Thomas, who was grandfather's brother:

> September 15, 1972
>
> "Dear Ceci:
>
> Sorry to hear that your Grandmother is 'failing' as we all do if we last long enough! I have been here about as long as I care to be – It has been so hard to come to this stage and place with nothing to look forward to – we can adjust when younger – This is a very lonely life but I have much to be thankful for."

Patients need to see more of their loved ones and friends…to be part of the world outside the nursing home. These nice people once had a life. They are human…and from my experience sweet, loving people. I asked a friend of ours why he hadn't visited Peter while he was at Hawthorne, as he had asked me out to lunch. He replied, "I hate nursing homes. I don't know what to say!" Why not try to say hello or how are you…your hair looks beautiful, or I like your pretty necklace…or don't say anything. Moreover, you'd be surprised how many family members could care less about their mothers, fathers, sisters, brothers, or friends once in a Home. I tried to lick this problem by getting to know and enjoy everyone each day I visited Peter. Marie, the ninety-four year old, whom I wrote about earlier, hadn't heard from her son since she moved in years ago. She would cry when she mentioned him. "We were so close. Why doesn't he come in to see me? My daughter comes some Sundays. She doesn't know why either."

I would also like to mention here that I tell my friends, who are couples, to enjoy each other's company as much as possible...make every day count...have fun, travel, do things together, for you never know what will happen tomorrow!

I quote a poem, "If I know," which I am fond of. Its author is unknown.

> "Hold your loved ones close today,
> Whisper in their ears,
> Tell them that you love them
> And you'll always hold them dear.
> For tomorrow is promised no one,
> Young and old alike,
> And today may be your last chance
> To hold your loved ones tight."

Since Peter's passing, I truly feel that I will be joining him in Heaven...his communicating with me has reaffirmed that there is life after death...that the soul leaves the body and transitions from Earth. I am convinced of this also after my accident and visit to Heaven. Peter's Spirit has been with me ever since his death. How? I have taught myself how to meditate and through mental telepathy have been able to reach Peter, or he with me. Ironically, each night for the first two weeks, in reaching him telepathically, when the love of my life appeared, my heartless, abusive father would intervene. Upon ignoring him, by addressing Peter by name over and over again, Daddy gave up and hasn't appeared since.

The night after my Husband's passing, I saw his dark figure kneeling at the side of my bed. This frightened me, as I let out a loud, "What?" He appeared for a moment and vanished...I think he was trying to thank me for taking care of him or tell me he loved me. Since then, I have begged him to give me a sign when he is present. I know I cannot see or touch him, but I can feel his energies. I asked him to let me know what he looks like, as he is now whole without Parkinson's...is he young, middle-aged, or the way he was when I last saw him? I now dream of my handsome, smiling, middle-aged Husband. When he is present, I feel a cold breeze across my path or a feeling of warmth when he is standing next to me. Frequently, I smell a familiar fragrance. Once when this happened, it led me to his bathroom. I went through his bottles of aftershave with no luck. I then came across his lip balm which he constantly used – that was the beautiful smell; moreover, had I not gone into that room, as the door was closed, I would not have found the dead ants that were all over the place. I think he was trying to steer me in that direction. Once up at "Thurtilperk Hill," our house in New Boston, I was in the bedroom. Lindsey was outside. Jen was lying on the bed asleep next to me. While I was reading, there were footsteps walking around the house – then the shade to a window in the living room snapped with a loud bang. Through mental telepathy I immediately told Peter and Anne, his late sister, to stop the trickery, as it was scaring me. I never experienced this again!

Sometimes I find "the raw emptiness," as I call it, and "the extreme, unbelievable loneliness" unbearable. Grief overcomes me. Peter was my companion, my best friend, my advisor, my lover, and my soul mate for fifty-four years. I miss taking care of him, his poule a la Hitchcock and cooking for him, traveling, entertaining, or just taking our daily walks together, much less snuggling with him. We were inseparable from the day we met, always doing and enjoying everything together, but I know now that what he is telling me is true..."We'll be together soon...we'll get through this...BELIEVE!" is helping me to live each day; however, Peter doesn't want me to grieve. He doesn't like it when I cry, but sometimes I have to let it out! Usually it's in the early mornings and at night I miss my Husband. I try not to be sad but sometimes I have to let go. Keeping in touch with each other has convinced me that there is more to life than on Earth. I quote from my Journal some brief messages Peter has given me:

1. I was crying – "I love you, Ceci," he said. "I love you, Peter," I responded. "You've got to go forward for us," he said. "But I want to join you, Peter," I lamented. "It's not the right time. Don't cry," he answered. "Don't do that. We'll be together soon."
2. "You'll be all right. We'll get through this," he said. Don't cry. I love you." "But I miss you," I sighed. "I'm here. I'm with you," said Peter. "You just can't see me."
3. One time when I was in a vicarious situation, I asked him to protect me from buckling. I'm with you, Ceci," he said. "You'll be o.k." I answered by saying, "I'm glad...why don't you call me Darling...you used to." "Sweet-Love, I'm with you...by your side," he said.
4. Coming back from New Boston on June 19, 2014, after driving bumper to bumper in heavy traffic, I left the Garden State Parkway, turning onto 195. Tears came to my eyes, as I approached the Jackson Exit. I

hated to go to an empty house without Peter. "Don't cry…please stop that," Peter said. "I can't help it. I miss you so much," I sobbed. "It's all my fault. I got sick with Parkinson's," he continued. "You have to wait. You'll be joining me later. Don't cry. We'll get through this. I love you." "I love you too, Sweetheart," I said. I felt at peace.

5. I had a dream of being with Peter, though I can't remember the particulars. As I was awakening with eyes closed, I said, "I miss you, Sweetheart." "But I've been with you all night," he laughed. "I know but it's not the same," I said. "I love you, my Darling," he responded. "Stay with me Peter…please…don't go," I begged. There was silence. I got up feeling at peace and dressed.
6. I woke up depressed and sad. I said to myself I should quit writing. I'll never get published. I heard Peter's voice, "No…no…no, Ceci. You're doing well. Don't give up. You can do it. What you've written is good." "I love you, Peter," I said. "Do you really think so?" "Yes…yes," he responded. "I love you, too."
7. I had finished typing a part of the Chapter, "The Proposal," one afternoon at four-thirty as I usually did, and put the television show, "Ellen," on. I looked up at the white tray ceiling of my bedroom and in black writing were the words, "I love you." I was shocked. Peter still had not told me he loved me, much less proposed to me.
8. Recently, I have received messages telling me that he is proud of "Same Time…Same Station." This has made me feel good as I have written it for him.

*****

Besides being able to communicate with Peter, I feel he is reaching out through flowers. I've had them year-round, especially at Christmas, on our wedding anniversary, Valentine's Day, and Easter. And much to my surprise, our Christmas Cactus, which must be at least twenty years old, going back to the Houston days, blooms every month of the year…whether it produces one flower or many it is always beautiful. The plant has never been repotted, though I have always added fresh potting soil once a year. Never has it bloomed this much. There are also several other houseplants that have bloomed unexpectedly.

Our rhododendron out front produced one flower, out of season, as did the azaleas. They would again bloom when the weather warmed up. Then in May when I drove up to "Thurtilperk Hill," I was welcomed with a sea of colorful flowers both in the meadow and around the outside of the house! They were everywhere; forsythia; one bloom on Anne's rhododendron in memory of Peter's late sister; lilacs, daisies, buttercups, and wild strawberries; irises bordering the stream; pink and white roses in memory of the Hitchcocks; yellow lilies, and so forth – never seen this early before. Butterflies flitted about from one flower to another on the pink laurels, as songbirds were in concert overlooking the fields and mountains, finding mates, raising the young, and hunting for food.

However, I found that the more I went up to New Boston without Peter, the more I felt uncomfortable being by myself in the woods, even though I had Lindsey and Jen. In the summer of 2014, we had a scary and annoying incident when a rabid skunk lumbered out of the woods around eight-thirty one night. It chased the dogs for an hour until Animal Control and the Chief of Police arrived to kill it. The dogs received boosters, and because I had scratches on my hands, I had to go through the series of rabies shots. That was the last straw. I had had enough of New Boston!

On April 1, 2015, I again put the house on the market. Two days later I received a bid from the novelist, Christopher Bollen, who had seen "Thurtilperk Hill" in 2013, commenting then that the property was "romantic," according to our broker. The closing was June 15th. I am overjoyed that the new owner wants to keep the ninety-two-year-old house the way it is, though, will probably have a larger kitchen built.

Needless to say, I miss "Thurtilperk Hill" but feel blessed, after fifty-six years, to have such wonderful memories. In fact, Christopher and I have kept in touch writing letters, mostly about how to run a seasonal home which he hopes to winterize. It is in good hands now. And my darling Husband has mentioned several times, through mental telepathy, that he is ever so proud of me for selling it to such a fine person, who will enjoy it as much as we did!

*****

In the near future, I have decided to move into a continuing life care community, living as an independent with my two dogs, Lindsey and Jen; moreover, I have begun to clean out the house on Oak Hill Court in Jackson, with the help of Sharon. In doing so I came across the many, many love letters I had slipped into Peter's briefcase when he traveled on business before his retirement. I was surprised to find out that he had kept them, but am thoroughly convinced of his devotion to me, as I have had with him. This has given me an amazing inner peace...a joyful feeling of being totally loved by my Husband for the fifty-four years we shared.

I quote one letter, a favorite during our twenty-seventh year of marriage:

> Sunday
> January 2, 1987
> "Peter Darling:,

Take care of my Sweet-Love. We were in such a hurry "doing everything" this morning before your flight that I want to say here: I, too, am glad I married you! (You touched me so by mentioning it.) I wish I could be in your pocket. I'm so proud of you because you are a great attorney. I love my Darling. And God bring you safely back to me.

Your Spoose"

No wonder we are in touch with each other telepathically. We are soul mates…a gift. Our love exemplifies the strong bond between us which we will have for eternity.

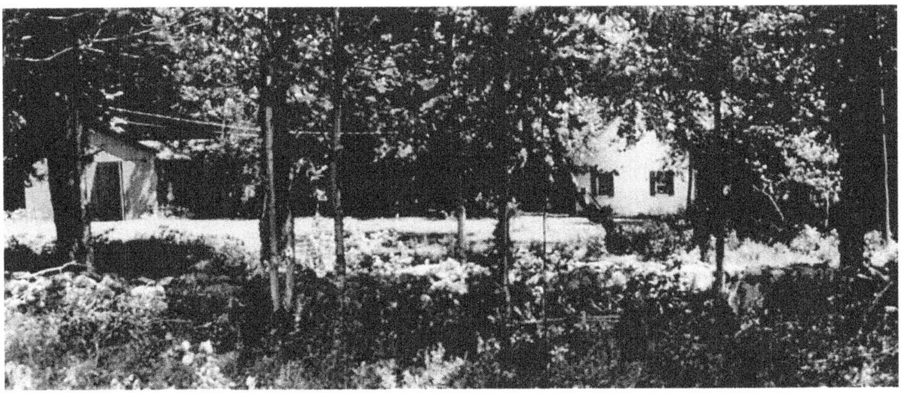

"Thurtilperk Hill" in New Boston, MA

# Acknowledgements

I would like to thank all those who helped me with "Same Time...Same Station;" their stories, wisdom, advice, encouragement, editing, and typing: Gail Shapiro, Jeanne Ogburn Barbour, Sharon Myers Hitchcock, Barbara Engler, Barbara Kohlsaat von Oehsen, Mike Morgan III, Starr Kohlsaat Hungate, Father H. Gaylord Hitchcock, Joy Farrar, and Bernadette Falcicchio Discon.

Made in the USA
Monee, IL
13 September 2026

62976394R00114